the bi(k)ini
competition
training
guide

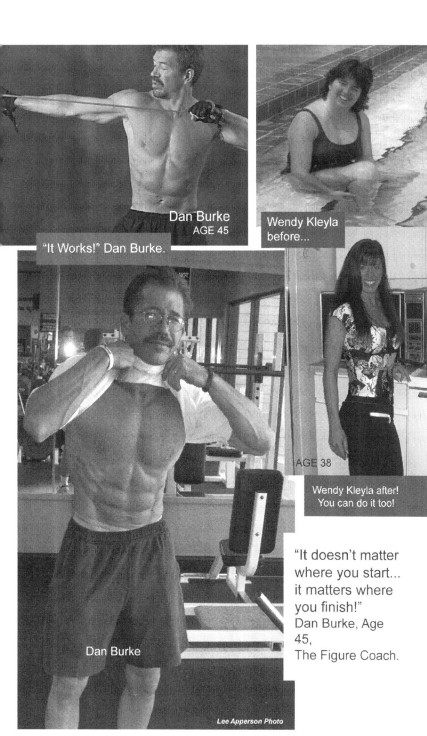

Dan Burke
AGE 45

"It Works!" Dan Burke.

Wendy Kleyla before...

AGE 38

Wendy Kleyla after!
You can do it too!

Dan Burke

"It doesn't matter where you start... it matters where you finish!"
Dan Burke, Age 45,
The Figure Coach.

Lee Apperson Photo

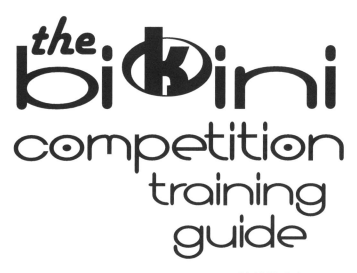

the bikini competition training guide

copyright 2010 Dan Burke

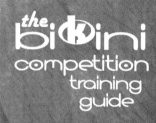

the **bikini**
competition
training
guide

Table of Contents:

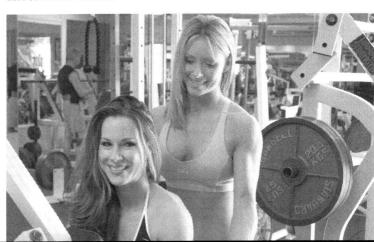

1. Introduction.

If you are new to training, allow about two years to get into contest shape. The average person can develop a great body in about 1-2 years, even with no prior training. If you have good genetics and are perhaps already athletic, it may take you less time to achieve a competition-ready body. Regardless of where you are starting from, our

common goal is to finish on stage, competing in a contest, looking like a living statue of a Greek Goddess in the winners circle. Getting in shape is never easy. It takes time and dedication to lean out and

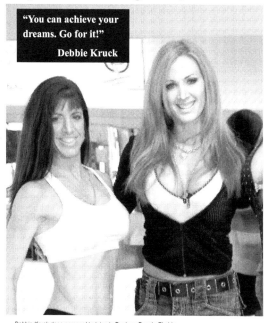

"You can achieve your dreams. Go for it!"

Debbie Kruck

Debbie Kruck does personal training in Daytona Beach, Florida.
(386) 566-3685 Call Debbie and go in for a workout!

exercise your way into a toned, super fit condition. As I said, it takes about one to two years for the average person to achieve a superb physical condition.

Then there is competing. Taking your body on the road to a stage and live audience and offering it up for the trials of woman vs woman competition. Competition is not for the faint of heart, and live competition is on another level all by itself. Being judged is harsh. But it will help you be subjective, and if you stick it out, become a champion. No one usually wins the first time out. We all make mistakes. We mature. But we also learn and adapt. Each time out we make a better game plan. If you devote yourself to becoming lean, and sexy, you will find yourself in the winners circle no matter where you place in a "contest".

This book is designed to help you become a female Bikini champion or just look like a champion. Bikini competitions are big business. Huge! From bathing suits, to shoes, to pro-tan, to contest hall rentals there are millions of dollars in the sport of being a beautiful female

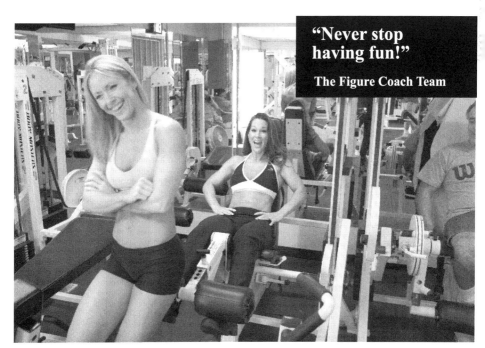

"Never stop having fun!"

The Figure Coach Team

athlete. What you do with your fame and fortune is up to you.

Guess what? We want you to win. We want you to experience everything sports, eating clean, training and striving to be 100% your best can do for you. It is a journey you will never forget. It will change you. You may surprise yourself along the way. Imagine being the best you can possibly be. Almost mind boggling. This book is the road map to that place. This book is your blueprint for success.

We often hold back from doing something because we don't have all the facts and the skills we need to be a success. If you want a sexy, fat free body, with a fit, feminine look, you are holding the right book in your hands.

This is your no nonsense success guide. You can look like a Bikini Champion if you follow the plan of action outlined in detail in this book. Yes, you can become a champion. All the tools you need to compete are here. The time, the desire, the hard work, that is all up to you. And sadly, no one can do it for you. Even movie stars can't hire someone to train—for them—but I know a few that actually tried it!

You can do it. Always remember that. The hard work will pay off. Will it take work? You bet! Is it worth it? You tell me. My answer is yes. For me, being fit and sexy brought me love, wealth and

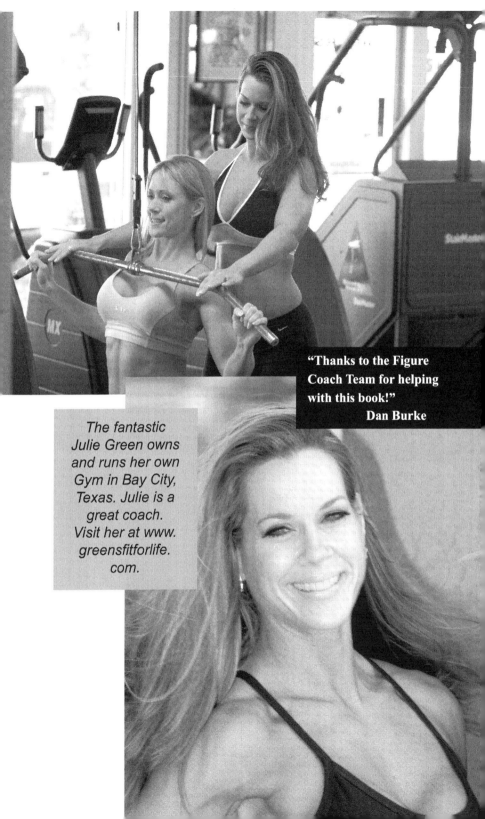

"Thanks to the Figure Coach Team for helping with this book!"
Dan Burke

The fantastic Julie Green owns and runs her own Gym in Bay City, Texas. Julie is a great coach. Visit her at www.greensfitforlife.com.

friendships that I cherish. Backstage at a show is a great place to meet your next best friend.

 Is looking like a living statue of female excellence something you are after? Are you wanting to walk around in a firm, feminine body that is both powerful and beautiful to behold? It's not for everyone. But if that is something you crave, you are on the right track.

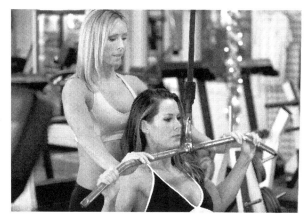

This book can help you compete and win. It can help you stay on track and develop a plan that will work for you. It can save you 1000 of hours of wasted time.

 We know that competing is exciting. The audience, the back stage rush, there is nothing like competing. Training normally is fun, but nothing and I mean nothing makes you focus on training and eating like the pressure of an approaching contest. It makes all the training and dieting count. It gives you a deadline to work towards. It helps you focus 100% on you.

Which is hard to do in this busy world.

No matter where you are you can achieve your fitness goals.

Everyone starts with nothing. At the beginning of any journey things can look difficult. More difficult than they really are. Take change one day at a time. And those days will add up!

Change is slow and can be painful. But you can do anything you set your mind to, that is a fact. You can change your life. You can change your body. Competing, dieting, and taking control of your body can be a catalyst for this change. Love yourself enough to trust in the process, never quit on yourself. Give yourself the gift of great health and a great body. If you are afraid, do not worry. It will pass. It doesn't matter where you start, it matters where you finish. Finish fabulous.

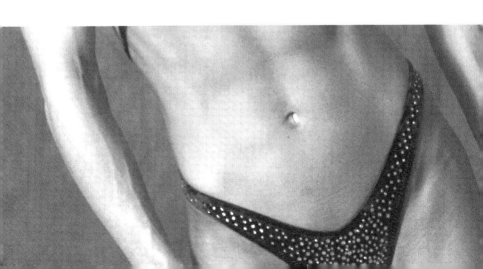

2. Bikini Competition.

Overview of competition:

Bikini is a modeling competition. You need a fit, firm, fat free, pleasing physique, with terrific tone, to compete in Bikini competition. You don't have to have breast implants nor do they count against you. Your entire body should be symmetrical. The contests are divided into tall and short class competitions. Also age groups, such as over 35, over 40, are also 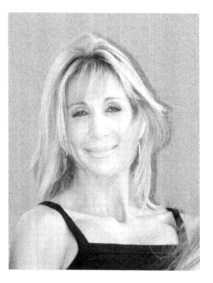 used to divide classes. How you walk, your hair, skin tone, face, all count in Bikini competition.

Bikini Competition is broken into 2 parts during actual staged competition.

1. Individual presentation. The athlete walks on stage and presents herself to the audience. Alone the athlete walks to the center stage and shows herself.

2. Direct comparison: Athletes are compared by the judges directly to one another. The competitors wear 2 piece traditional bikinis and high heels. They are compared in 2 poses: front pose and back pose, standing. There is no flexing of muscles.

These both occur (individual presentation and comparison rounds) at the morning prejudging or evening prejudging. What is prejudging? This is the time when the real contest happens and the judges score the athletes. The evening show, or main show is when the audience comes to watch and the awards are presented and the overall winners are chosen.

So you have to be prepared to both walk and present yourself and compare to others in a line up.

What to expect if you win your class. Let's say you win the tall class at your contest. You would then return to the stage and be

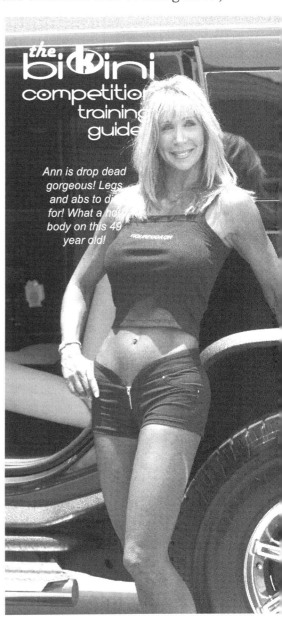

Ann is drop dead gorgeous! Legs and abs to die for! What a hot body on this 49 year old!

compared live in front of the audience, against the short class winner and an overall winner would be chosen.

If you do not win your class you do not compete for an overall title.

You can wear a different bathing suit, jewelry and so on for the prejudging than you might wear for the night show. You can also wear the same suit if you choose.

What will you need to win? That is what this book is all about.

Mastering your Individual presentation:

The competitor walks on stage to the center. She stops and does her front pose or position. Always with a smile and a positive attitude. How you walk,

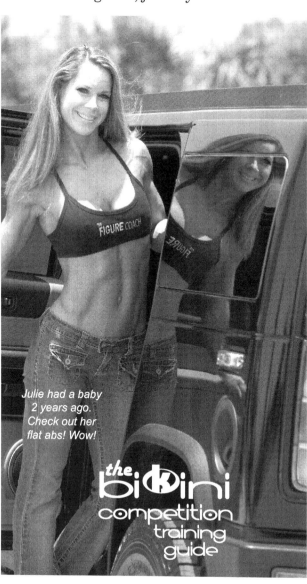

Julie had a baby 2 years ago. Check out her flat abs! Wow!

the bikini competition training guide

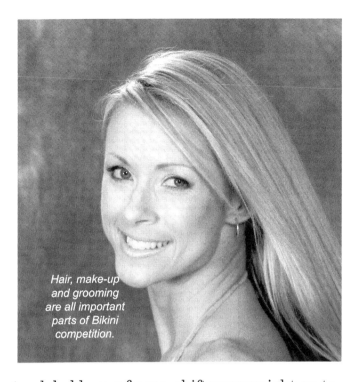

Hair, make-up and grooming are all important parts of Bikini competition.

stand, hold your frame, shift your weight on to one foot, all is part of your presentation. Then you turn. If you are good you do a smooth turn or pivot turn. The competitor turns to the rear and again pauses and holds a pose. How you stand is up to you. But usually a tilt or accented leg stance is used to make the athlete look good.

We present good examples of standing poses that you can learn from and create variations. You only have a few seconds on stage so here is some advice.

1. Walk slow. Much slower than you think you should. Your stage walk is so important that you should have practiced it for months. It should be sexy but not comical. Relaxed and confident. Head and chin up. A slight bounce is okay.

2. Smile at the judges and audience. Radiate personality. Keep your head up.

3. Have great hair and make up to match your body. Your face and body should all be the same color. Special attention should be paid to your hair.

4. Bathing suit. This suit should be a solid color and fit like a glove. 2/3's of your buttocks and breasts should generally be covered. No micro suits. Cut the strings off your suit to a short length. The suit can make or break you, so it's very important you get a suit that fits correctly on you. I suggest getting a custom made suit to fit perfectly. The suit should be smaller, not bigger. Looking sexy and fit is the goal.

5. Shoes. 3 inches is fine. You don't have to go higher. Color match your suit if you can. Your shoes should be tasteful and something you can walk in easily. Practice walking in shoes for many hours before you compete on stage. Practicing and perfecting a good stage walk is essential.

6. Turns and standing. How you stand and turn is a key part of Bikini Competition. You need to nail this and do it right every time. No time for being shy or looking awkward. Again, you need to practice your stands and turns till

they come very naturally. And yes, smile as you turn and stand. Head up, body arched, neck and hands relaxed.

Comparison Rounds: Direct comparison to others in your class.

This is where you are directly compared to each athlete. Head to head as individuals. You walk to the center stage and get in a line up. Each athlete stands to the front. Then they are asked to turn to the rear. They do so and then stand. This takes place usually 2 or 3 times. Often athletes are moved in the lineup so all the judges can see each athlete. Try to relax here and smile. All your training is about this moment.

What is in it for me to become a Bikini athlete?

You will notice that to become successful at Bikini competition and other athletic sports takes work. A ton of work. Like most things that do not come easily or without effort there is an entire set of traits, habits and other things, that develop because of the task.

Working for a goal teaches people that they can achieve things they desire by hard work and dedication. It teaches them the 1,000 mini-lessons that add up to one big lesson. The ability to develop confidence and greater health, a better body and self image are just a handful of things training for bikini competition and creating a great body can do for you. The obvious thing about a Bikini competitor is that she is beautiful. Great hair, great make up, great legs. But what people can't see is all the WORK it took to GET that way.

We know that your appearance effects the world around us. Guess what? The world effects us too! Living life as we suggest, eating clean, exercising daily, resting, grooming and so on, will lead you on a life path that will amaze you. And will alter HOW OTHER PEOPLE TREAT YOU.

A big part of that journey will be competition. Getting on stage and putting it all on the line and competing against others. Win or lose.. competing changes a person. Striving for a goal creates something GOOD in people and it will do so in you! Let's take a look at just a handful of the amazing benefits of devoting yourself to a long term goal like Bikini competition that promotes clean eating and healthy living.

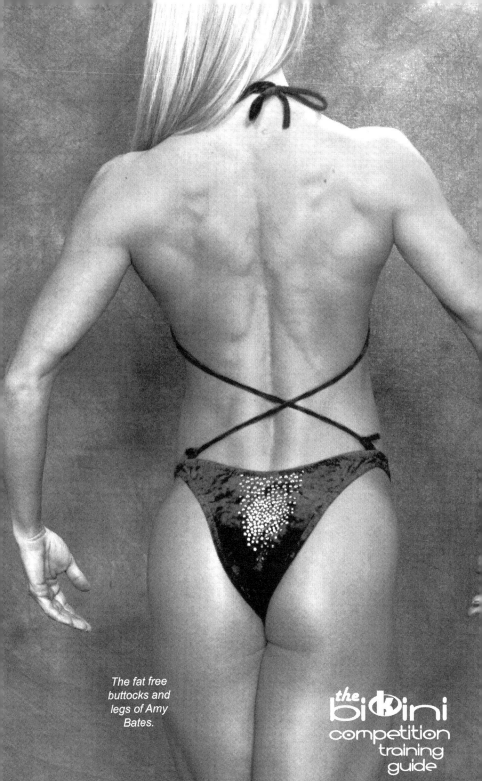

The fat free buttocks and legs of Amy Bates.

the
biƉini
competition
training
guide

3. Benefits of Bikini Competition.

1. Poise and physical balance.

2. Learning to strive for a goal.

3. Better health and physical well being.

4. Resistance to illness.

5. Deeper and more restful sleep.

6. Greater self confidence, and mental focus.

7. Stronger heart, muscles and lungs.

8. Increased ability to handle large crowds and appear on stage. Stage presence is developed.

9. A healthier, stronger, sexier body.

10. Increased attractiveness to others. Possible modeling work, meet possible mates and more.

11. Decreased body fat.

12. Develop friendships with like-minded people.

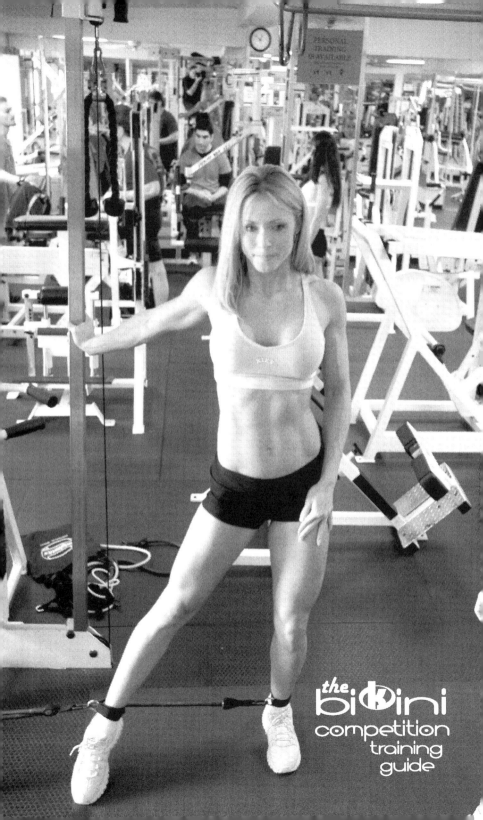

the bikini
competition
training
guide

4. The NPC Bikini rules.

HEIGHT CLASSES – For Pro qualifying event

Up to and including 5'1"
Over 5'1" and up to and including 5'2-1/2"
Over 5'2-1/2" and up to and including 5'4"
Over 5'4" and up to and including 5'5-1/2
Over 5'5-1/2" and up to and including 5'7"
Over 5'7
If promoter chooses to do fewer height classes:

For all contests with two (2) classes:
Up to and including 5'4"
Over 5'4

For all contests with three (3) classes:
Up to and including 5'4"
Over 5'4" and up to and including 5'6"
Over 5'6

For all contests with four (4) classes:
Up to and including 5'2"
Over 5'2" and up to and including 5'4"
Over 5'4" and up to and including 5'6"
Over 5'6"

COMPETITOR RULES

National level contests do not permit competitors to crossover into Bodybuilding, Fitness or Figure at the same event. All other competitions are permitted to have crossovers at the discretion of the promoter with district chairperson approval. Competitors will compete in a two-piece suit. The bottom of the suit must be v-shaped. No thongs are permitted. Competitors can compete in an off-the-rack suit. All swimsuits must be in good taste.

Competitors must wear high heels.

Competitors may wear jewelry.

COMPETITION JUDGING

Presentation

Competitors will walk on stage alone and perform their Model Walk (personal preference)

The Model Walk consists of the following:

Walk to the center of the stage, stop and do a front stance then a full turn and do a rear stance then turn to the front again in front of the judges and then proceed to the side of the stage.

Comparison Round, Two-Piece Swimsuit

Competitors will be judged wearing a two-piece swimsuit and heels.

The competitors will be brought out in a group and directed to do a full front and rear stance. Judges will have the opportunity to compare competitors against each other in half turns. (No side judging permitted, front and back only.)

Judges will be scoring competitors on the following items:

Balance and Shape

Overall physical appearance including complexion, skin tone, poise and overall presentation.

REVIEW: The NPC is not the only sanctioning body for Bikini contests. The rules are different for each organization so be sure to get the rules before you decide to compete.

The NPC is a national sanctioning body and a great place to compete. You have to pay to compete in the NPC sanctioned contests. Other established contests like Miss Hawaiian Tropic, Hooters and others actually are free to compete in and give out cash prizes. Where you compete will be up to you. Your bathing suits, tan, body are an investment and you should be entitled to make money from all that hard work.

5. Competition Waivers:

Open competitions, for cash or not, can be a great place to practice your stage presence. The downside is that these unsanctioned shows often take place in places that allow alcohol drinking. This changes the tone of the contest. It can quickly deteriorate into an ass shaking contest in front of a screaming drunk crowd which you want to avoid. Where you compete is up to you and you need to feel safe. Often when you compete you sign a waiver which allows the promoter to use the photos and video footage of the event as they see fit. This is an important consideration. Sometimes a high profile show, like Hooters, can be a great place for exposure. If you do not want your image showing up in the wrong place or even the right place out in public, be sure to investigate and read the competition waiver carefully. Sometimes missing a contest is not a big deal if you may be photographed at that show and those photos can be sold without your consent.

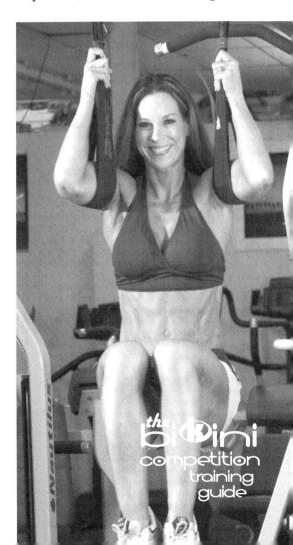

6. Your Plan of Action.

You will be breaking your training into a yearly cycle. If you are new to training, you will find that each yearly cycle leaves you in better shape. The yearly cycle has 4 seasons: Spring: Break-In Training. Summer: Peak Training. Fall: Peak for a show. Winter: Rest.

Once you are in shape you can jump into peak training almost whenever you want. You can do a string of shows over a years time, peaking for each show. This is a successful plan of action used by millions of athletes. It works for them and it will work for you. Periods of intense effort require periods of rest or injury and sickness and

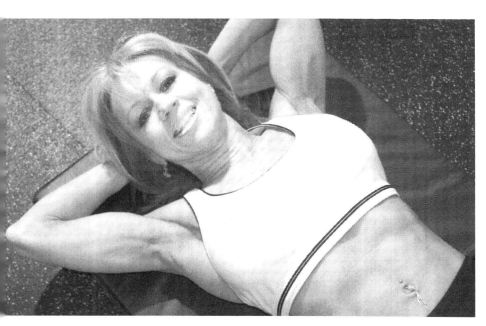

decreased performance will develop.

For beginners you need to focus on mastering the peaking process and getting in great shape without injury or wasting valuable time.

The goal is to get yourself in better shape gradually, over 12 months, dieting and training harder as you approach the end of the year, your contest or goal.

To start the year, you focus 3 to 4 months on conditioning and losing fat. Work out but not too hard. Then 3 to 4 months on training hard to firm up and really get off more fat. This is followed by 3 to 4 months working to a peak, achieving a "peak" condition.

After that, 3 months of "active" rest. Train-

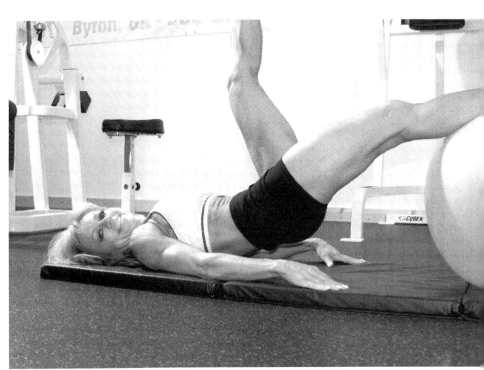

ing, as before, but not as intensely. Many athletes follow even longer cycles. They spend years working on building up, or fat loss, till they are ready to go to the next step. I trained almost daily for 12 years before I competed for the first time. You have to pay your dues. With hard work the average person can build a great body in just a year or two.

A yearly cycle is a good idea for athletes. It

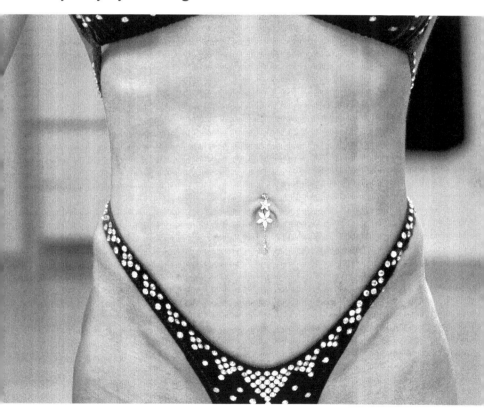

stops you from burning out and allows your injuries to heal.

Most of how you look will be determined

by body fat levels and diet. Great training will not replace or make up for lousy dieting that makes you fat. Try to stay in decent shape all year. That way, when it's time to compete, you only have to diet for several months to get in "top shape". If you can't see your abs, you are too fat. Some fat, like the fat on our butt cheeks or lower back, that accumulates with age, seems to defy all dieting and workout techniques. You train and train and diet and it just sticks there. Will it come off? The answer is "yes", but you have to stick with it. The fat will come off, but it will take time.

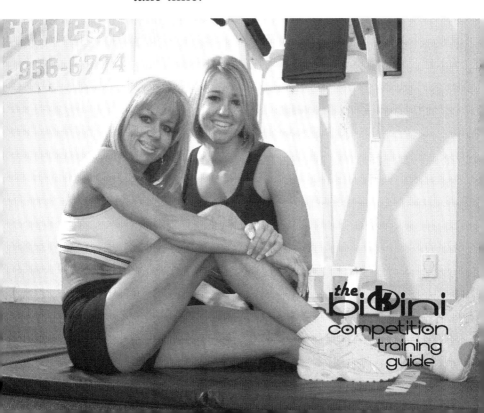

7. The Yearly Shape Up Plan.

So let's take a detailed look at your plan of action. Go get a calendar and make notes. Split the year into 4 parts and make a goal for each part of that plan.

Plan your SUPER HARD training time (maybe the summer), then plan your "off season" training time (maybe the fall). Look at the year as a whole unit of time and break it into 4 parts.

It's important that you start looking at training in the BIG picture and train towards specific goals.

Allow time for rest and recovery. Do not attempt to be training and dieting hard all year. You need a break. Rest is as important as training.

If you are fat, your overall goal no matter what yearly phase you are in is to lose fat. Till that happens that is the goal. Once the fat is gone (year two) you may find yourself focusing on more body training with weights as part of your overall yearly training goal. As you progress your personal goals will change. As you age, you will find the challenges to get in shape, year after year, changes as your body ages.

Always plan your year with an OVERALL goal for the YEAR, and create a goal for each training phase.

winter

What to do:
Heal injuries. Focus on conditioning and weak points. Do not lift heavy.

How to train and eat:
Weights: 2 to 3 workouts a week. Full body workouts. Avoid training injured parts. Diet at 80%.

spring

What to do:
Ramp up training. Perform cardio full time if needed, and lift weights with a serious mind. Train your weak points all the time.

How to train and eat:
Weights: 2 to 5 workouts a week. Split routine. Focus on fat loss and getting stronger. Diet at 95%.

summer

What to do:
Training is full bore now. Building up and training hard. Cardio is full time.

How to train and eat:
Weights: 5 to 10 workouts a week. Split routine. Focus on getting in top shape. Diet at 99%.

fall

What to do:
Hit a peak. Cycle in from the summer. A six to twelve week sprint to the contest. After competing, rest for several weeks. Then engage in 2 months of light training.

How to train and eat:
The 6 to 12 week peak. Train all the time and eat clean. Pose every day. Diet at 100%.

8. The 4 phases.

PHASE 1
4 months off season.

Easy training.
Heal injuries.
Diet at 75%.
Cardio part time.

PHASE 2
4 months strength training.

Hard training.
Focus on weak points.
Diet at 85%.
Cardio part time.

PHASE 4
4 months competition training.
Building to a peak and then competing.
Hard training.
Focus on Peak training and losing all body fat. Diet at 100%.
Cardio full time.

PHASE 3
4 months competition training.
Hard training.
Focus on total body look.
Diet at 95%.
Cardio full time.

No matter what the yearly phase keep in mind these 3 levels of interest.

Master posing, walking on stage, makeup, and grooming. Plan to compete in multiple shows to really become polished and poised on stage. Practice posing daily for months before competing.

1

Train with weights consistently. Train progressively. Plan to break up your training into split training sessions so you can focus on different body parts.

2

Perform fat burning or cardio exercises every day or even 2x each day (till the fat is gone). Walk or ride a bike, do aerobics of any sort at a pulse rate of about 115 to 125 beats per minute for 30 minutes 1 to 2x every day.

3

Your 12 month plan:

Months 0 to 3:

Cardio exercise.
Fat burning exercise 3 to 5 days a week.

Weight training. Full body training for 3 months.

Dieting. If you are fat, time to get it off. If you are thin and weak, try to focus on eating lots of good food and building yourself up.

Months 4 to 6:

Cardio exercise.
Fat burning exercise 5 days a week.

Weight training. Split training. Each body part 2x a week.

Dieting. If you are fat, keep dieting. If you are thin and weak, focus on eating lots of good food and building yourself up.

Months 7 to 9:

Cardio exercise.
Fat burning exercise 5 days a week. Double cardio (2 sessions a day) may be needed.

Weight training. Split training. Each body part 2x a week. Workouts are about peaking now. You can train more frequently to increase definition.

Dieting. Contest diet. 12 to 16 weeks or less of clean eating to get your bodyfat down to nothing.

Months 10 to 12:

Cardio exercise.
Fat burning exercise may stop if you are fat free. You should be fat free by now. If not keep doing cardio. Focus on weight training to peak yourself. If you are still fat--**keep doing cardio** till the fat is GONE.

Weight training. Split training. Each body part 2x a week or more. Intense effort is applied at this time.

Dieting. Contest diet. Diet ends when you compete. Return to regular eating after you peak and win your contest. Rest Injuries after competing, train light.
Recover.

10. Starting from zero.

Not all of you..but some of you, may find yourself in no physical condition at all. Maybe you had a baby, or just took a few years off from exercise after college. The reason is not important. What you do next is important. No matter how it happened, you have not exercised in years, and you are starting at "physical" ground zero.

So for those that need the advice we will talk about strategies to use when your body is in no shape at all to exercise. Consult a Doctor to make sure you are healthy enough to exercise.

1. Most important, do not injure yourself. Always under-do it, rather than over-do it.

How do you avoid injury? Do NOT train until you are sore, tired, or become "shakey". Do NOT do things that overly stretch or contract you. Use light weights, with careful smooth movements. Move slowly and carefully when you perform exercises.

2. Give yourself several weeks or months to break into "full time" training.

For those that can do it the idea of small workouts spread throughout the day works great. This avoids becoming overly tired at any one time. Rather than one long hour workout, four 15 minute workouts, spread out throughout a single day, can help a beginner, do a complete routine without becoming overly tired. Here are some specific examples of this sort of training:

Beginners one week sample:

Beginners One day split:

Monday am:	10 minute bike ride.
Monday am:	10 min. weight training.
Monday pm:	10 minute bike ride.
Monday pm:	10 min. weight training.
Tuesday	Rest.
Tuesday	Rest.
Wednesday	Rest.
Thursday am:	10 minute bike ride.
Thursday am:	10 min. weight training.
Thursday pm:	10 minute bike ride.
Thursday pm:	10 min. weight training.
Friday	Rest.
Saturday	Rest.
Sunday	Rest.

This is a good example of how to train for short periods through the day and week and slowly expand your limits. More people can endure 10 minutes of exercise several times a day rather than one long training session. It works great for people that are just beginning to exercise after a long break. It avoids becoming overly tired or sore.

11. Fat Loss and Fat Burning.

Losing fat is a large part of getting in great shape. Sometimes that is all it takes to look great. Once the fat is gone your natural shape and tone can show. Using exercise as a sculpting tool, you can make your waist smaller, your legs more shapely, your butt round and so on. A layer of fat, that hides natural shape and muscle tone, is something we do not want, and much

of our time as athletes may be devoted to the single task of losing unwanted body fat. Bikini competition does not require you to diet down to some super low body fat. Nothing like a body builder, marathon runner

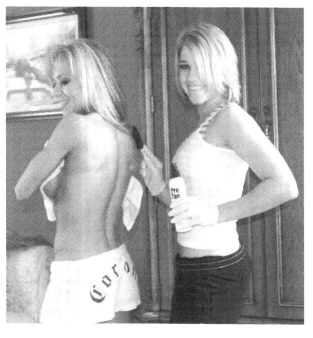

or some other extreme sport. You need fat, a small amount of it, to look healthy and full. You need a normal full (not scrawny or too thin) looking body that is healthy and toned looking. Having some fat, as a female, looks good. You do not want to diet to the point of being too thin, or underfed looking. A full, robust body, even if you are 5' 2" and weigh 98 pounds is what you are after.

In the following section we include a plan of action for eating right, choosing the right foods, and then putting it all together into a daily diet plan.

Are you an athlete? Is a model an athlete? For our purposes anyone interested in using Bikini as a competition platform is an athlete. You have a goal in mind and you are trying to look your best.

Fat accumulates according to genetic pattern on our bodies. Each person is different to a point. Your butt may be your primary fat storage area or your arms or your lower stomach. Where you store the fat first (on

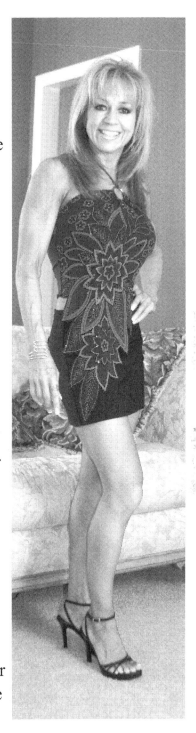

me it is my stomach) is where you tend to lose it the last.

Fat Loss Targets: These are the areas that are going to give you the most cause for concern. Often one area just will not let the fat go. You diet down till you look thin and slim but this one part of you just holds onto the fat! Sound familar?

This is normal. Plan on adding 2 months to your fat loss schedule to fight off that last 5 pounds. The last 5 pounds, which seems to always stick like super glue to a target area, is the hardest to lose for many people.

The body is fighting you, trying desperately to hold onto this fat and not let it go! Only at the end of the diet will this fat come off. It's difficult and takes great effort but it will happen.

Be aware of your fat loss targets. Put your time into these target areas and lose the fat!

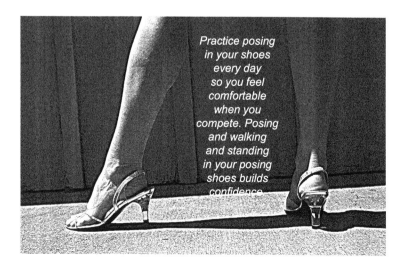

Practice posing in your shoes every day so you feel comfortable when you compete. Posing and walking and standing in your posing shoes builds confidence.

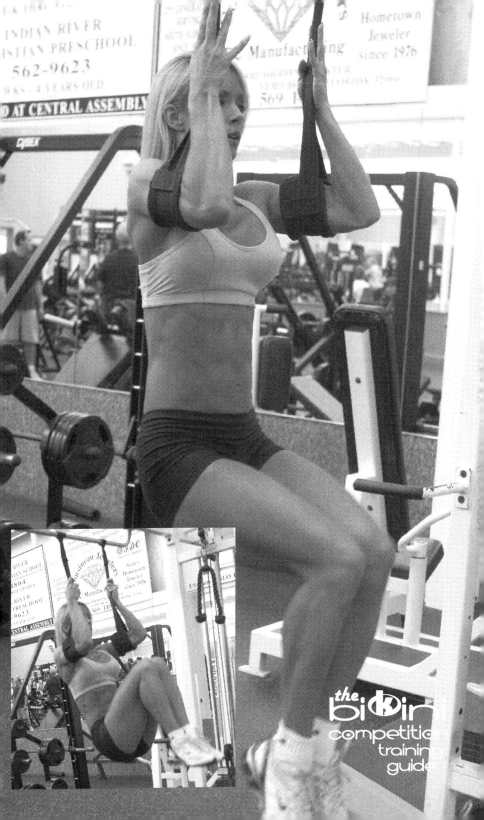

12. Fat Loss Targets.

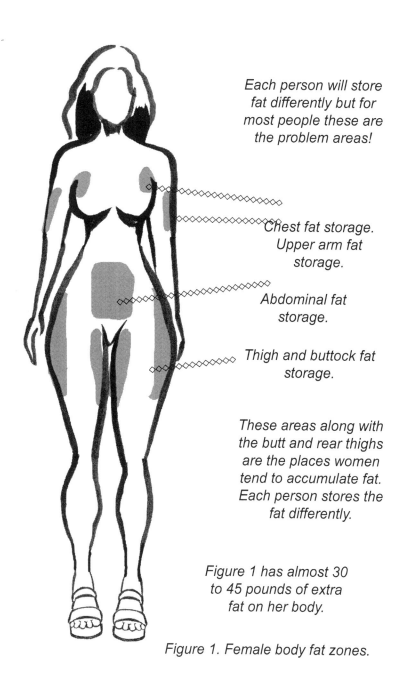

Each person will store fat differently but for most people these are the problem areas!

Chest fat storage.
Upper arm fat storage.

Abdominal fat storage.

Thigh and buttock fat storage.

These areas along with the butt and rear thighs are the places women tend to accumulate fat. Each person stores the fat differently.

Figure 1 has almost 30 to 45 pounds of extra fat on her body.

Figure 1. Female body fat zones.

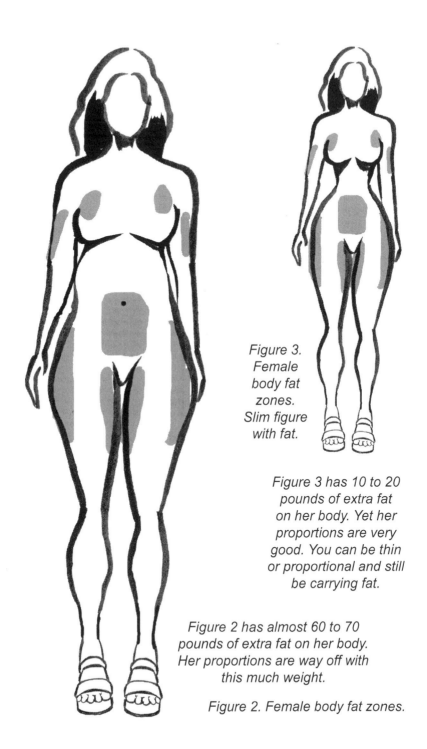

Figure 3. Female body fat zones. Slim figure with fat.

Figure 3 has 10 to 20 pounds of extra fat on her body. Yet her proportions are very good. You can be thin or proportional and still be carrying fat.

Figure 2 has almost 60 to 70 pounds of extra fat on her body. Her proportions are way off with this much weight.

Figure 2. Female body fat zones.

13. Fat Loss Timeline.

Great expectations is what we should all have for ourselves when it comes to shaping up. It can be done. It comes down to eating and exercise and time. Time is the tricky part of the story because when it comes to fat loss, time seems to move ever so slowly.

I will put a disclaimer that says results may vary on this chapter, but based on my 30 years of training people I can safely guess as to how long it takes to lose fat for many individuals.

There are several ways to look at this equation. But let's delve into simple math, focusing on the sum of the formula: E x E,

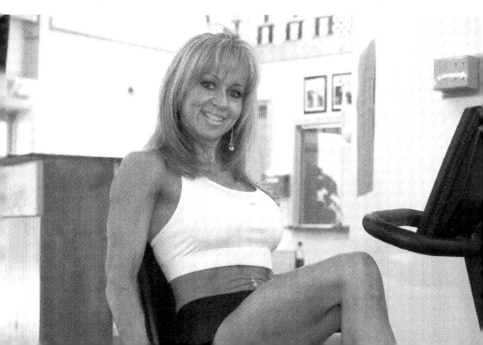

divided by T, equals your result. Eating x Exercise divided by Time equals results.

First we will define what we mean by "eating".

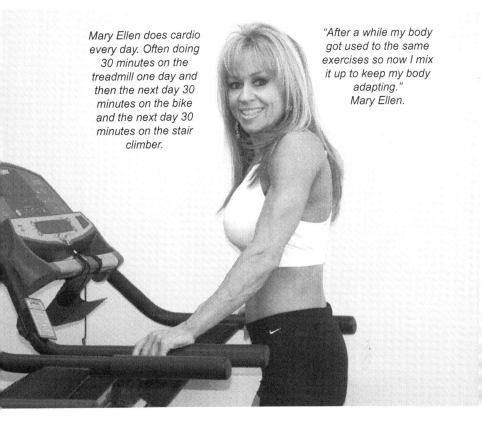

Mary Ellen does cardio every day. Often doing 30 minutes on the treadmill one day and then the next day 30 minutes on the bike and the next day 30 minutes on the stair climber.

"After a while my body got used to the same exercises so now I mix it up to keep my body adapting."
Mary Ellen.

We mean clean eating, without eating junk of any kind. You can eat a ton of clean food, but clean food only. That is the "E" of our formula.

Then we go to exercise. Exercise, the second "E" in the formula, is defined as 30 to 40 minutes fat burning cardio sessions

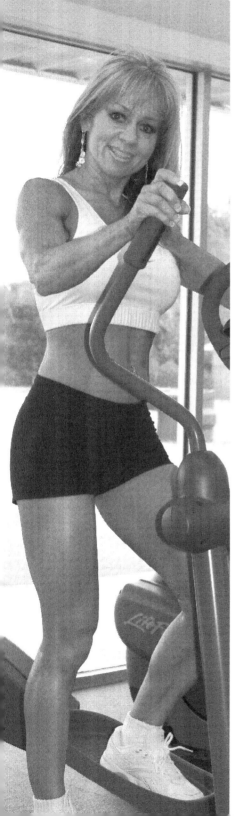

daily.

Those two things along with time yield the following results:

If you are doing 25 cardio sessions a month (this is based on taking 5 days off per month to rest, and training the other 25 days) and eating clean, expect to lose 5 pounds of fat a month.

Can you lose more? Can you lose less? Maybe. But for 90% of those reading this you can safely expect to lose 5 pounds every 4 weeks.

This is not always reflected on the scale as an exact 5 pounds, but you will be shrinking and getting smaller.

So over 4 months you can expect to lose 20 pounds of pure fat if you keep the program running as described.

I have noticed that the longer you continue eating clean and exercising to burn fat (as in months) the faster the progress gets.

There is a marked difference in performance and fat loss for most individuals comparing month one 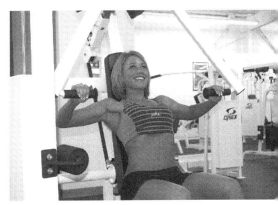 versus month three or four. In other words the longer you train and diet, the better you become at losing fat.

Most people who eat clean and exercise for 6 months lose 45 pounds of fat. For some people that is half a person! You are thinking hey that is MORE than 5 pounds a month. And the fact is, this has been my experience with dedicated and focused individuals.

These are reliable estimates for you to bank on for your fat loss program.

14. Losing the last 5 pounds.

We talked earlier about stubborn body fat and that losing the last 5 pounds of fat from our frame is difficult. The last 5 pounds seems to stick like glue and often to one area of our body. How do we get rid of that last 5 pounds? Why is it so hard to get rid of? What strategies can we use to rid ourselves of this last unwanted 5 pounds of fat?

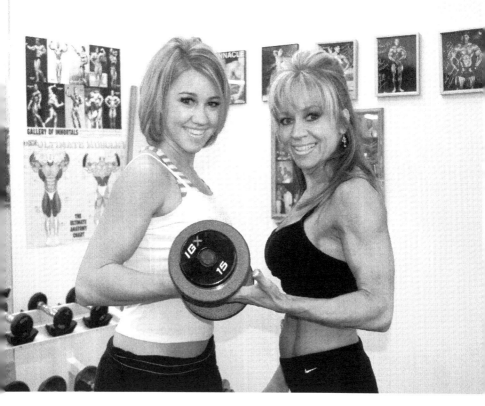

The body needs fat. It wants fat. Fat is your body's protection from starvation. Your body will often use up (for energy) muscle or other tissue rather than burn fat tissue. The body hoards fat. It makes it fast, and is slow to give it up. As we get lower in bodyfat our body sort of warms up to the task and really gets things going. But as we get to 10% or below in bodyfat level, the body begins to fight against any further loss. It gets worried that maybe there may be a famine and that the body could die, so it holds onto the last 5 to 10 pounds of fat like life depended on it.

But don't worry, for a bikini competitor a super low bodyfat level is not needed. Being firm and fat free is the look you are after. That is about a 10 to 12 percent body fat for most bikini competitors.

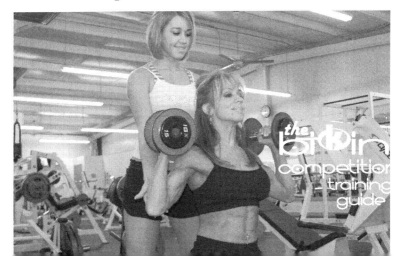

5 pound loss strategies:

1. Plan on dieting super strict for 4 to 8 weeks. Keep a diary.

2. Do not starve yourself. Eat clean food only and eat a lot of it. Eating more, as long as it's clean and you are active, won't make more fat.

3. Increase exercise. Do fat loss or cardio training 2x a day for a total of ten, 30-40 minute sessions, every week. That is 40 cardio workouts in 4 weeks! This is a lot of increased activity and combined with eating clean, has a **big impact on body fat levels.**

4. Eat every 3 hours. Keep your blood sugar level constant to avoid dips in blood sugar. 6 small meals a day or more for 4 to 8 weeks.

5. Lift weights or some sort of resistance training 3 times a week.

6. Carb and protein rotation. For 3 days eat a high protein diet with little carbs, then on day four, have a high carb day. Keep this rotation going. You can also do this one day protein, one day carbs, but it seems to work better with a several day rotation. Here are some examples of protein/carbohydrate rotation diet days:

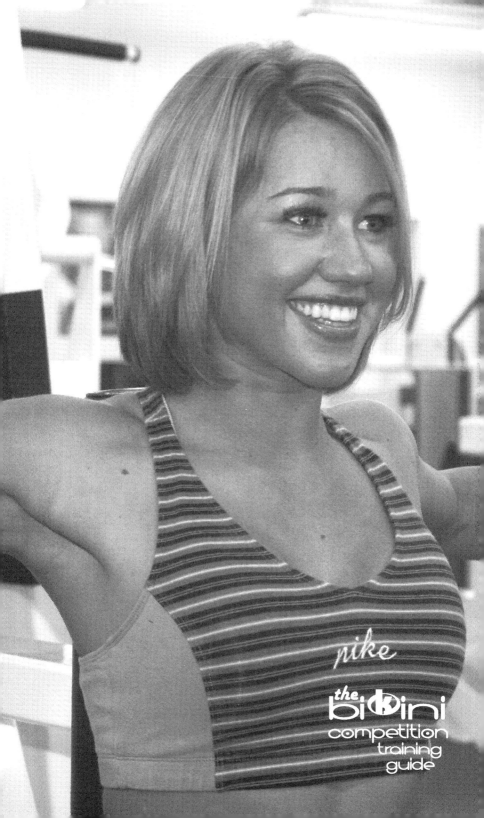

nike

the biԿini
competition
training
guide

ROTATION DIET:

Example one:

DAY ONE: High protein.

DAY TWO: High protein.

DAY THREE: High protein.

DAY FOUR: High carbohydrates.

Example Two:

DAY ONE High protein.

DAY TWO High carbohydrates.

DAY THREE High protein.

DAY FOUR High carbohydrates.

Example three:

DAY ONE: High protein.

DAY TWO: High protein.

DAY THREE: High carbohydrates.

DAY FOUR: High protein.

DAY FIVE: High protein.

DAY SIX: High carbohydrates.

7. Prescription fat loss drugs. You need a medical

doctor to help you with this one. A fat loss specialist MD is best.

In essence you take a prescription drug that speeds up your metabolism. These work in a variety of ways and beyond the scope of this book. How do you know if you need it or can obtain it? Call you doctor and make an appointment. Have your thyroid checked and make sure your glands are working correctly.

Even if you are healthy you may be a candidate for prescription drugs that help with fat loss. Often a diet specialist doctor can prescribe medications that can speed up your metabolism and accelerate fat loss without danger. The drugs are never to be used without a doctor's direct involvement. Never self-prescribe medication. Side effects can be sleeplessness, and other problems. So the benefits have to be weighed against the negatives. However, these drugs are powerful and they work.

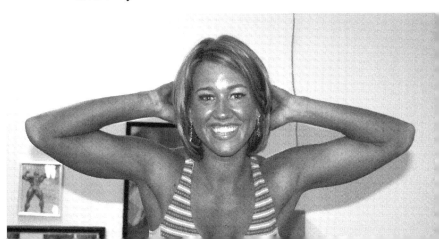

15. Shopping for fat loss.

Your shopping list:

1. 2 pounds chicken breast.
2. 2 pounds fish.
3. 1/2 pound lean filet to grill.
4. 10 to 25 pieces any fruit, including:
   5 oranges.
   5 peaches.
   5 apples.
   6 bananas.
   4 pints berries.
5. Salad mix (low calorie dressing). 5 servings of salad.
6. Low-fat cheese.1/2 pound.
7. 2 sweet potatoes.
8. 4 cups brown rice.
9. 4 ears of corn.
10. 5 bags of frozen vegetables.
11. Skim or soy milk.
12. Choose 5 fresh vegetables. Buy 2 servings of each.
13. 5 gallons fresh water.
14. 1 cup low-fat cottage cheese.
15. Nuts. Dry roasted.
16. 1 dozen eggs.
17. Seasonings for fish and chicken. Choose as many as you enjoy.

Ingredients to make protein shakes:
1 container of whey protein.
1/2 gallon non-fat milk, soy milk or water.
Frozen mixed berries, 16 oz.
Non-fat, sugar-free ice cream or frozen yogurt.
Fresh or frozen fruit of all sorts.

Throw away the junk food in your home. You can always buy more and get fat later. Now it's all about eating clean and getting lean and sexy. To keep it simple we have laid out the foods you want to look for when you go shopping. 3 to 4 servings of clean carbohydrates a day and the same with proteins. It's a simplified way to look at eating but it works. Should you count calories? It can't hurt. Keeping a food journal can be a valuable step in getting organized in your eating. When you go to the store to shop, you need to only buy good food that contributes to your goals.

Workout Dairy:

To really get an accurate view of your eating you really need one of these. It allows you to keep accurate track of your training program and food consumption and slowly reduce calories in small increments by reducing 100 calories a day. Only by keeping a journal can you truly gauge the results of a pattern of eating and how that directly affects your body's fat levels. All beginners should keep a training diary for the first year at least. The best competitors keep a journal FOREVER. Frank Zane, Bill Pearl, Lee Apperson, and others, including your author (I have training journals since I was 12 years old) all use them. In my mind you can't make REAL progress without one. If you are competitive weight lifter, a record log is imperative. You have to learn to cycle your training and "peak" with your strength. Keeping a training journal is the ONLY way to do this accurately.
Workout Dairy. One final thought: it keeps you honest with yourself about your workouts and how many calories you are consuming.

16. The rules to losing fat.

The Rules of Losing Fat:

1. Do cardio (fat burning) exercise 5x per week or more.

2. Weight train 1 or 2x per week or more.

3. Eat 3 pieces of fruit a day.

4. Triple the vegetables. 3 small servings at every meal.

5. Drink a glass of water before each meal.

6. Don't confuse tiredness with hunger.

7. Do nothing else when you eat. No TV or distractions.

8. Cheat smart. Reward yourself ONLY when you've REALLY earned it.

9. Prepare your food ahead of time and carry it with you.

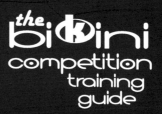
the bikini competition training guide

10. Do not eat past 7:30 - 8:00 at night. Do not snack in the evening.

11. Do not skip meals or become too hungry.

12. Eat small servings.

13. Eat frequently. Carry good food with you at all times.

14. Eat "net negative" calorie foods, foods high in fiber like celery and salad.

15. Burn more calories than you take in. Generally eat around 1,200 - 1,500 calories everyday.

16. Never starve yourself by skipping meals.

17. Don't drink calories. No juice, soda, or alcohol.

18. Do not purchase or eat junk food.

19. Get your proper rest. Take naps if you can. Daily cardio is taxing on your body.

17. The clean food list.

Suggested Food List:

FRUITS
Apples
Apricots
Bananas
Berries
Cantaloupe
Grapefruits
Lemons
Mangoes
Oranges
Peaches
Pears
Pineapples
Plums
Watermelon

VEGETABLES
Beets
Broccoli
Cauliflower
Carrots
Celery
Collard greens
Corn
Cucumber
Dark green leafy lettuce
Green peas
Kale
Kidney beans
Lima beans
Onions
Red and green peppers
Romaine lettuce
String beans
Sweet potatoes
Spinach
Squash
Tomatoes
Zucchini

PROTEIN

MEATS (*3 to 6 oz.*)
Chicken breast
Lean beef
Turkey breast

SEAFOOD
Clams
Crabs
Fish (all kinds)
Lobster
Oysters
Shrimp

EGGS
Egg whites

MILK AND CHEESE
2 cups non-fat milk
2 cups soy milk
5 oz. low-fat yogurt
4 oz. low-fat cheese
Non-fat sour cream

Suggested Food List:

PROTEIN

AMINO ACIDS
BEEF
BROWN RICE/BEANS
(combined)
CHICKEN
DAIRY PRODUCTS
(low-fat)
EGG WHITES
FISH (all types)
LAMB
LENTILS
LOW-FAT YOGURT
MILK, CHEESE (low-fat)
PORK
PROTEIN POWDERS
SHELLFISH
(clams, crab, lobster,
oyster, shrimp)

SOY
SOY MILK
TOFU
TURKEY

CEREALS and GRAINS
Bran flakes
Brown rice
Corn flakes
Puffed rice
Puffed wheat
Whole wheat

SPICES
Garlic
Oregano
Pepper
Salt
Sea salt
Thyme

DRINKS
Water, tea, coffee
Lemonade (made with real lemons and sugar substitute)
Whey shakes (low calorie, high protein)
Zero calorie drinks

LIST OF FOODS NOT TO EAT OR DRINK:

Alcohol
Bacon
Bread/muffins/bagels
Butter
Cakes
Candies
Canned fish in oil
Canned fruit in syrup
Canned vegetables in oil
Cookies and crackers
Doughnuts
Fast food
French-fries
Fried food (all kinds)
Honey
Hotdogs
Ice cream
Juices
Lattes and frappuccinos
Pork/ham/sausage
Potato chips
Smoothies
Sodas
Sugar
White flour products
White potatoes
White rice
Whole milk and cheese
Yogurts (whole fat)

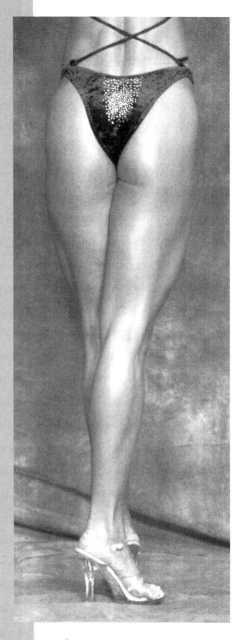

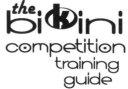

the bikini
competition
training
guide

18. The daily eating plans.

Making it all work.

Knowing what to eat and when to eat it is more than half the battle. Your activity level will determine how much you need to eat. If you are hungry, eat. If you are eating clean you can eat quite a bit and not become fat. When exercising you will find your metabolism increasing along with your appetite. That is okay. Eating small meals of clean food throughout the day (literally eating all day long) is fine as long as it's clean food.

Not eating food that replaces or creates MORE fat is a very important step for your weight loss.

Eating clean food, even large amounts of it, will not make you fat. Junk food makes you fat. Bread, sugar and alcohol make you fat. Carrots, apples, even if you ate a dozen of them every day for years on end, would not make you fat.

Follow the sample diets. You can eat the same food choices over and over if they suit you. Make small modifications to the daily plans as needed, they are not written in stone.

If you are not losing fat fast enough do not starve yourself, rather **increase activity.**

DAILY EATING PLANS 1

Meal 1

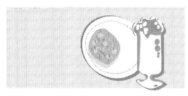

Oatmeal. Protein shake.

Meal 2

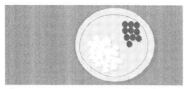

Cottage cheese (low-fat). Grapes.

Meal 3

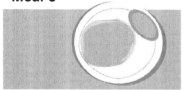

Grilled Salmon. Sweet potato.

Meal 4

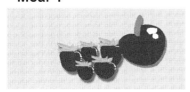

Apple. Berries.

Meal 5

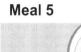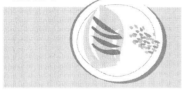

Grilled chicken. Wild rice (1/2 cup).

Meal 1

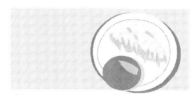

Cheese omelette. Orange.

Meal 2

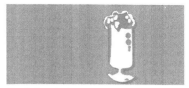

Protein shake.

Meal 3

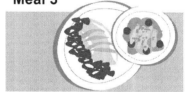

Chicken with tomato sauce. Salad.

Meal 4

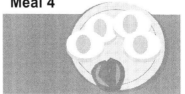

Hard boiled eggs. Peach.

Meal 5

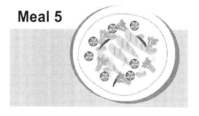

Chicken stir-fry with mixed fresh vegetables.

DAILY EATING PLANS 2

Meal 1

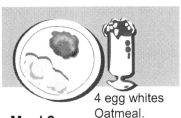

4 egg whites
Oatmeal.
Protein shake.

Meal 2

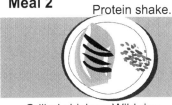

Grilled chicken. Wild rice (1/2 cup).

Meal 3

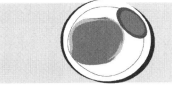

Grilled fish steak. Sweet potato.

Meal 4

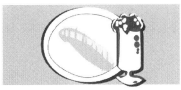

Baked fresh fish. Protein shake.

Meal 5

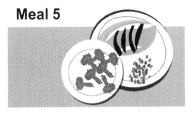

Grilled chicken.
Wild rice (1/2 cup). Broccoli.

Meal 1

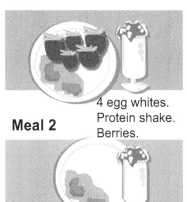

4 egg whites.
Protein shake.
Berries.

Meal 2

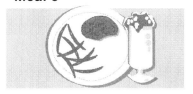

Protein shake. 4 egg whites.

Meal 3

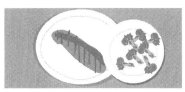

Grilled steak. String beans. Protein shake.

Meal 4

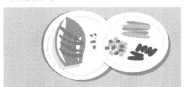

Baked fresh fish. Broccoli.

Meal 5

Grilled chicken.
Wild rice (1/2 cup). 3 vegetables.

DAILY EATING PLANS 3

Meal 1

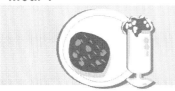

Oatmeal. Protein shake.

Meal 1

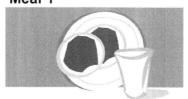

Protein pancakes. 8oz. skim milk.

Meal 2

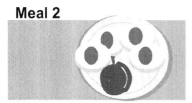

Hard boiled eggs. Apple.

Meal 2

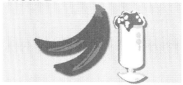

Protein shake. Fruit.

Meal 3

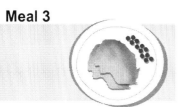

Turkey breast. Peas.

Meal 3

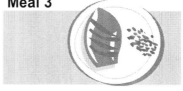

Grilled chicken. Wild rice (1/2 cup).

Meal 4

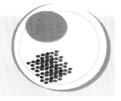

Sweet potato. Brown rice (1/2 cup).

Meal 4

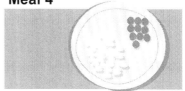

Cottage cheese (low-fat). Grapes.

Meal 5

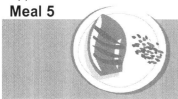

Grilled chicken. Wild rice (1/2 cup).

Meal 5

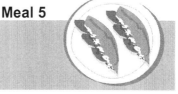

Lettuce wrapped fajitas. Non-fat sour cream, tomatoes, lettuce and salsa. Grilled chicken, shrimp or steak.

SNACKS

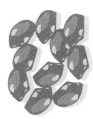

Sugar-free jello.

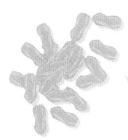

Unprocessed nuts of all sorts (dry roasted).

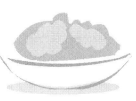

Sugar-free, fat-free ice cream or ice-milk.

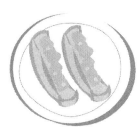

Celery with 3 tablespoons of all natural peanut butter.

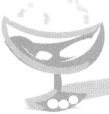

Low-fat yogurt.

Banana protein pudding. Whey protein blended with skim milk, sugar-free banana instant pudding, and a banana.

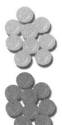

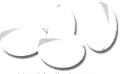

Hard boiled eggs.

Frozen Grapes.

Carrot sticks.

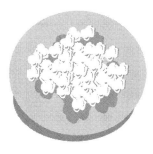

Popcorn (plain, air-popped) 2 cups.

DAILY EATING PLANS 4

Meal 1

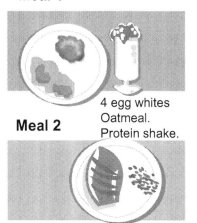

4 egg whites
Oatmeal.
Protein shake.

Meal 2

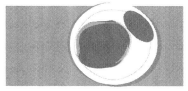

Grilled chicken. Wild rice (1/2 cup).

Meal 3

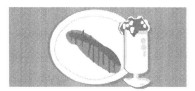

Grilled fish steak. Sweet potato.

Meal 4

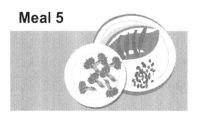

Baked fresh fish. Protein shake.

Meal 5

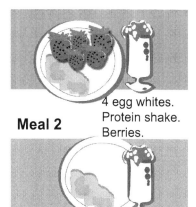

Grilled chicken.
Wild rice (1/2 cup). Broccoli.

Meal 1

4 egg whites.
Protein shake.
Berries.

Meal 2

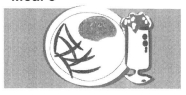

Protein shake. 4 egg whites.

Meal 3

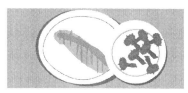

Grilled steak. String beans.
Protein shake.

Meal 4

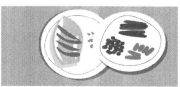

Baked fresh fish. Broccoli.

Meal 5

Grilled chicken.
Wild rice (1/2 cup). 3
vegetables.

High Protein Days

Meal 1

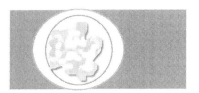

Meal 2

9 egg whites.

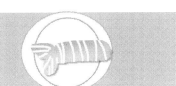

Lobster tail. 6 oz.

Meal 3

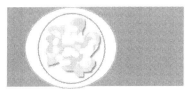

9 egg whites.

Meal 4

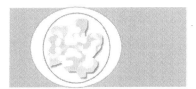

9 egg whites.

Meal 5

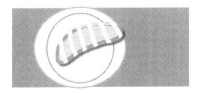

Grilled fish. 10 oz.

Meal 1

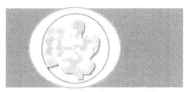

Meal 2

9 egg whites.

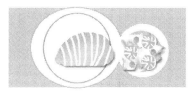

Grilled chicken. 6 oz.

Meal 3

Raw salad.

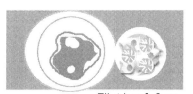

Filet beef. 6 oz.

Meal 4

Raw salad.

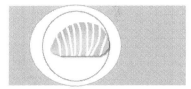

Grilled chicken. 6 oz.

Meal 5

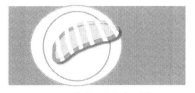

Grilled fish. 10 oz.

High Carbohydrate Days

Meal 1

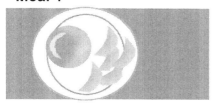

Peach slices. Grapefruit.

Meal 2

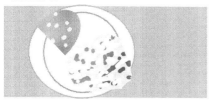

Brown rice.
Half sweet potato.

Meal 3

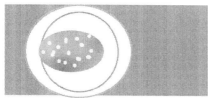

Whole sweet
potato.

Meal 4

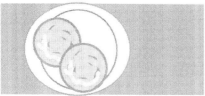

Whole wheat pancakes.
Sugar free syrup.

Meal 5

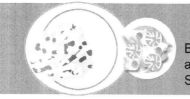

Brown rice with nuts
and corn.
Small raw salad.

Eat any of these foods:
Alfalfa Sprouts
Artichoke Hearts
Arugula
Asparagus
Bamboo Shoots
Bean Sprouts
Beet Greens
Bock Choy
Broccoli
Brussels Sprouts
Cabbage
Cauliflower
Celery
Celery Root
Chard
Chicory
Chives
Collard Greens
Cucumber
Dandelion Greens
Eggplant
Endive
Escarole
Fennel
Hearts of Palm
Jicama
Kale

High Carbohydrate Days

Meal 1

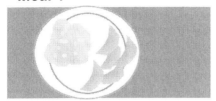

Oatmeal. Orange slices.

Meal 2

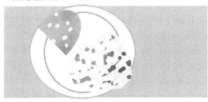

Brown rice.
Half sweet potato.

Meal 3

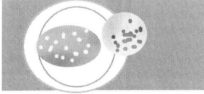

Whole sweet potato.
Orange.

Meal 4

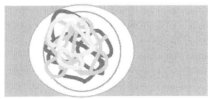

Whole wheat noodles.

Meal 5

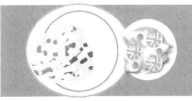

Brown rice with nuts
and corn.
Small raw salad.

Kohlrabi
Leeks
Lettuce
Mache
Millie lettuce
Mushrooms
Okra
Olives
Onion
Parsley
Peppers
Pumpkin
Radicchio
Radishes
Rhubarb
Sauerkraut
Scallions
Snow Pea Pods
Sorrel
Spaghetti Squash
Spinach
String beans
Summer Squash
Tomato
Turnips
Water Chestnuts
Wax beans
Zucchini

DAILY EATING PLANS 5

Meal 1

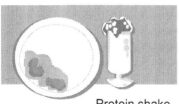

Protein shake.
6 egg whites.

Meal 2

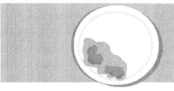

6 egg whites.

Meal 3

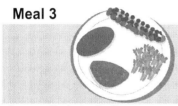

6 oz. grilled steak. Corn.
Broccoli. 1/2 sweet potato.

Meal 4

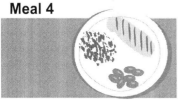

Baked fish. Mexican rice (1/2 cup).
Lima beans.

Meal 5

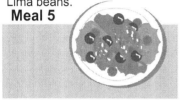

6 oz. grilled chicken breast with
fresh greens, tomatoes, walnuts,
and cucumbers.

Meal 1

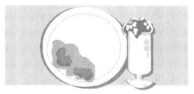

Protein shake. 6 egg whites.

Meal 2

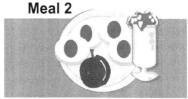

Hard boiled eggs. Apple.
Protein shake.

Meal 3

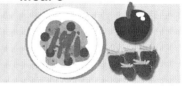

Vegetable salad. Fruit.

Meal 4

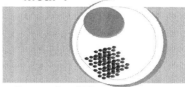

Brown rice (1/2 cup).
1/2 sweet potato.

Meal 5

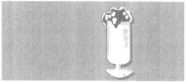

Protein shake.

DAILY EATING PLANS 6

Meal 1

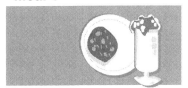

Oatmeal. Protein shake.

Meal 2

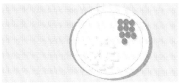

Cottage cheese (low-fat). Grapes.

Meal 3

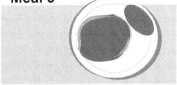

Grilled Salmon. Sweet potato.

Meal 4

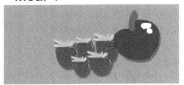

Apple. Berries.

Meal 5

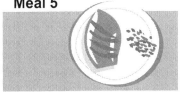

Grilled chicken. Wild rice (1/2 cup).

Meal 1

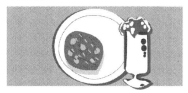

Oatmeal. Protein shake.

Meal 2

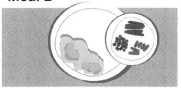

6 egg whites. 3 vegetables.

Meal 3

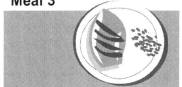

Grilled chicken. Wild rice (1/2 cup).

Meal 4

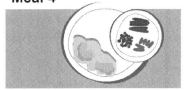

6 egg whites. 3 vegetables.

Meal 5

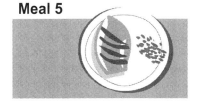

Grilled chicken. Wild rice (1/2 cup).

DAILY EATING PLANS 7

Meal 1

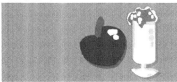

Apple.
Whey protein shake.

Meal 2

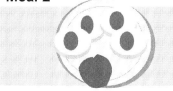

Hard boiled eggs. Any fruit.

Meal 3

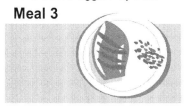

Grilled chicken (4 oz.). Wild rice (1/4 cup).

Meal 4

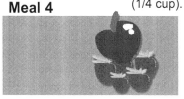

2 servings of any fruit.

Meal 5

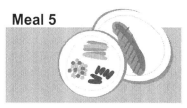

8 oz. of grilled fish.
Assorted steamed vegetables.
Peas, green beans, and carrots.

Meal 1

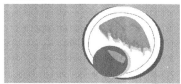

Cheese omelette.
Orange.

Meal 2

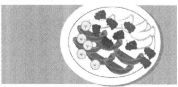

Fruit salad. Berries, apples, bananas, tangerines.

Meal 3

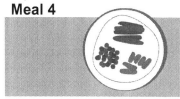

Hard boiled eggs.
Any fruit.

Meal 4

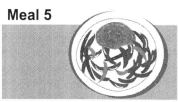

3 servings of any vegetables.

Meal 5

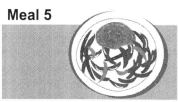

Breaded in corn flakes and oven roasted, chicken or fish with roasted vegetables. Add fresh green beans.

DAILY EATING PLANS 8

Meal 1

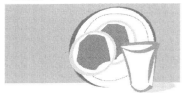

Protein pancakes. 8 oz. skim milk.

Meal 2

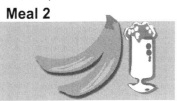

Whey protein shake.
Fruit.

Meal 3

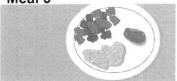

Mixed berries, 1 oz. dark
chocolate and protein pudding.

Meal 4

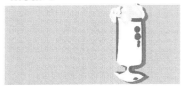

Protein shake.

Meal 5

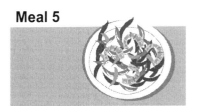

Stir-fry shrimp and
vegetables.

Meal 1

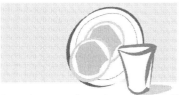

Protein pancakes. 8 oz. skim milk.

Meal 2

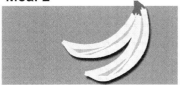

Fruit.

Meal 3

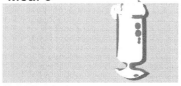

Protein shake.

Meal 4

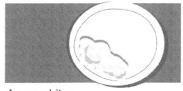

4 egg whites.

Meal 5

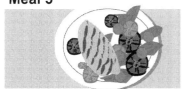

Jerk grilled chicken on a bed of
greens, tomatoes, and cucumbers.

DAILY LOG

Keeping track of your eating and training can help you stay motivated and stay on target. As your muscle tone and strength increase, your waistline and head-to-toe body fat will decrease.

BEFORE	AFTER
Paste Your Picture Here.	Paste Your Picture Here.

BEFORE   **AFTER**

BODY WEIGHT:	
WAIST MEASUREMENT:	

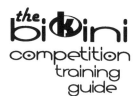

DAILY LOG

CALORIES

MEAL 1

MEAL 2

MEAL 3

MEAL 4

MEAL 5

CALORIE TOTAL:

BODY WEIGHT: WAIST MEASUREMENT:

| AEROBIC TRAINING | SESSION 1 | TIME: |
| | SESSION 2 | TIME: |

RESISTANCE TRAINING

EXERCISE	SET 1	SET 2	SET 3
1 WEIGHT REPETITIONS			
2			
3			
4			
5			
6			
7			

19. Posing and presentation.

POSING:

How you present yourself is an important part of competition. There are guidelines and rules you need to adhere to which help bring structure to the contests.

STAGE WALK:

It is painful to watch a women walk in heels who has NO IDEA how to walk in a pair of heeled shoes. You have to focus and practice. No one is born knowing how to walk on tiny platforms. You have to practice.

Practice daily on a hard surface:

For at least 3 months before your contest practice walking for a few minutes a day. Practice your entire routine. Walk, stop, pause, stand for several minutes in one spot and practice turning. Practice, practice, till you can walk very naturally in your shoes.

STAGE WALK RULES:

1. Avoid a marching or walking with legs bent.

2. Walk with your head up and shoulders back.

3. Put a slight curve into your lower back and keep your chest up.

4. Walk slowly but not too slow. Never fast.

5. A slight curve to your hips is okay. Not too much. Do not bounce as you walk.

6. Arms should move as you walk.

7. Hands should be relaxed and not tense.

8. Smile.

9. Glue your suit in place so you can ignore it.

10. Make sure your shoes fit.

11. Practice your turns. You can pivot turn or simply step and turn or both. However you turn try to keep it natural looking.

12. Walking when viewed from the back: Keep the head up. Do not lean forward. Shoulders should be up and back. Push your chest forward. Walk slowly.

13. Do not look down while walking or standing. Make it a habit not look down at your feet or the floor anytime while competing.

Stage walk: Cross step.

Walking correctly: The Cross Step technique.

You place one foot in front of the other as if you are walking along a thin line or rope in front of you. As you walk each foot is placed on that single thin (imaginary) line.

The feet have to cross the body (inwards towards the center of the body) as you walk in order to walk this imaginary tight rope. Watch models on a run way. Their feet criss-cross as they step, with the toe slightly pointing out. This is natural and shifts the hips as you step. This can be overdone, so you have to practice to make it look natural.

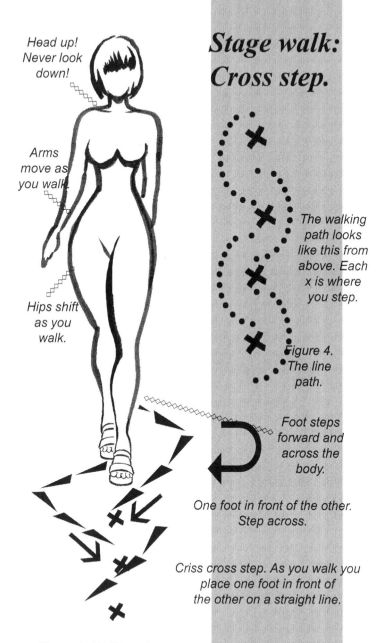

Stage walk: Cross step.

Head up! Never look down!

Arms move as you walk.

Hips shift as you walk.

The walking path looks like this from above. Each x is where you step.

Figure 4. The line path.

Foot steps forward and across the body.

One foot in front of the other. Step across.

Criss cross step. As you walk you place one foot in front of the other on a straight line.

Figure 3. Walking the line.

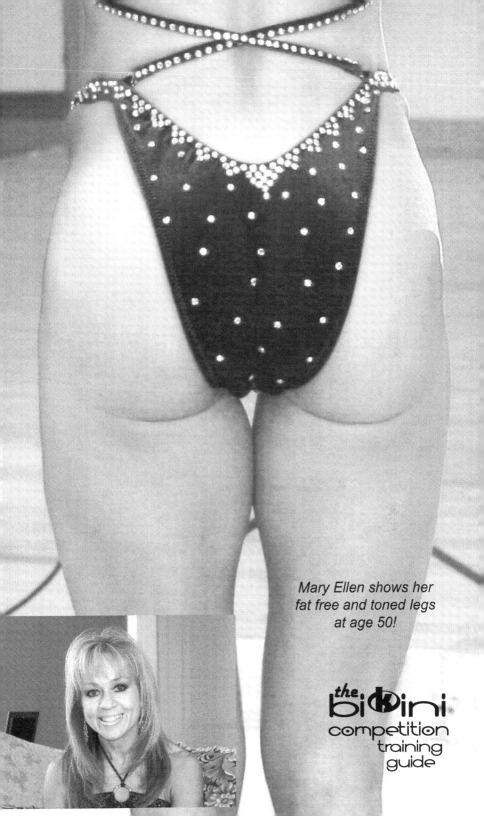

Mary Ellen shows her fat free and toned legs at age 50!

the bikini
competition
training
guide

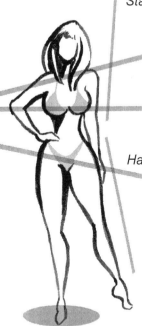

Stand straight.

Weight axis.

One shoulder lower..one higher.

Hand on one hip. Tilted weight.

Hands relaxed.

Hip tilted and accentuated.

Figure 5.

Leg straight.

Foot to side and hyper extended.

Weight on right leg and leg straight.

Weight axis.

Lower shoulder and higher shoulder. Notice tilt of upper torso.

Arm straight in front of leg or behind.

Hand on hip.

Figure 6.

Weight is tilted through hips. Weight on one leg.

Leg to side and straight as shown. Foot to side.

Weight on right leg and leg straight.

Leg creates this shape.

Elements of stage presentation:

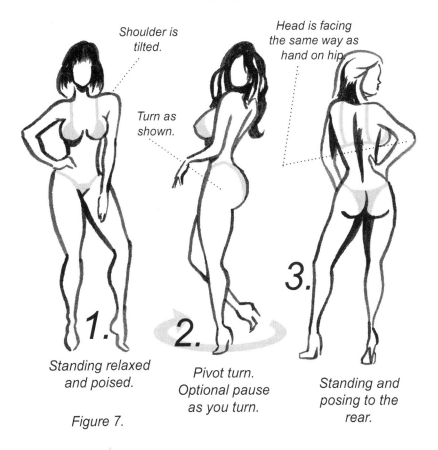

Shoulder is tilted.

Head is facing the same way as hand on hip

Turn as shown.

1. Standing relaxed and poised.

Figure 7.

2. Pivot turn. Optional pause as you turn.

3. Standing and posing to the rear.

After stage walk, how you present yourself in one spot is broken into 2 parts. **Turning and standing, to the front and back.** The **front pose** is a true model pose. Held for a second or two, you should look relaxed. You can shift from right foot to left foot and shift hands. Smile. Head and chest up. You may find tilting or turning your head slightly to favor your face structure is a good idea. There are many variations of a model stance. Choose one that is comfortable for you. Do not bend the legs, straight legs look better.

1. Pivot **turn.** Bring feet together and rotate smoothly. You can step behind the front foot (closest to audience) and pivot on the front or back foot.

2. Standing to the rear. Tilt the pelvis forward and push out your buttocks. Arch your lower back slightly here. You can stand straight or tilt the hips, to the side (see Figure 8) one hand on one hip displacing the weight onto one leg. Look over your shoulder and smile. Hand on hip on the opposite side you turn your head. Figure 9 shows this pose.

Weight balance:

Putting your weight onto one leg and holding a pose is not as easy as it looks. In figures 8 to 11 we see the basic stances that you should master. Failing to get your weight correctly balanced will cause you to look awkward.

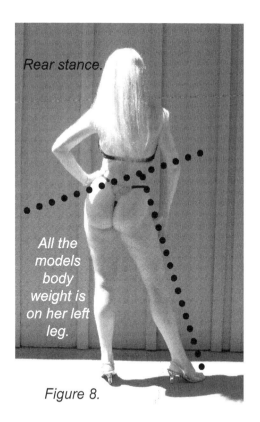

Rear stance.

All the models body weight is on her left leg.

Figure 8.

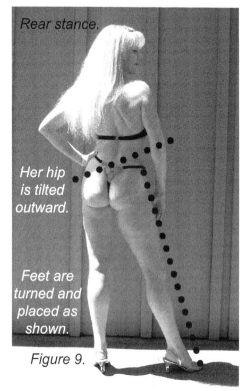

Rear stance.

Her hip is tilted outward.

Feet are turned and placed as shown.

Figure 9.

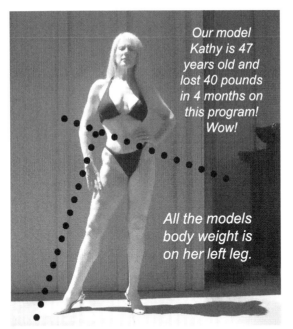

Our model Kathy is 47 years old and lost 40 pounds in 4 months on this program! Wow!

All the models body weight is on her left leg.

Front stance.

Figure 10.

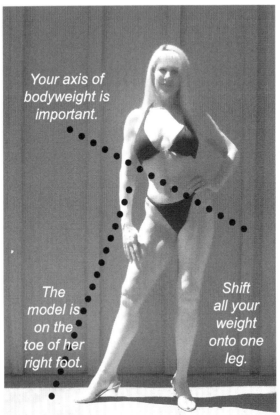

Your axis of bodyweight is important.

The model is on the toe of her right foot.

Shift all your weight onto one leg.

Front stance.

Figure 11.

20. Foot stances in detail.

Looking good on stage takes practice. How you place your feet will determine your balance and how you are perceived by the audience and judges. You want to stand the best way you can to show your figure to it's best advantage.

You want to practice your stances months and weeks before your contest. Practice is essential. Don't try to   just wing it. Take photos. Practice before a mirror. Find the poses that work best for you. Based on your structure (bone and muscle) you will find some poses that really work great for you and others that don't. Posing is open to interpretation. Make the best of it.

Standing in the lineup while other people pose. Often after you present yourself you will find yourself standing off to the side while still on stage. Be sure to stand perfectly while others present themselves and keep smiling. Never look down, fidget, scratch an itch and display other odd stage behaviors. Remember you are always competing till the contest is over--always look good on stage.

There are wrong ways to stand. Anyway that makes you look awkward is the wrong way to stand. Take photos and video of your rehearsals.

Now let us take a detailed look at standing starting from the ground up. That begins with shoes that fit and placing the feet correctly.

Standing correctly:

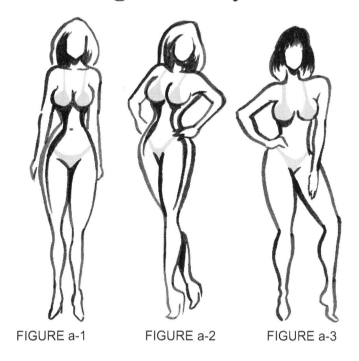

FIGURE a-1   FIGURE a-2   FIGURE a-3

FIGURE a-1:

Do not stand like this in your contest. Even when you think no one is looking. Even just turning sideways would be better than a full on stiff military pose like this. Do not stand like this.

FIGURE a-2:

This is not bad especially if you are totally relaxed. It could be a good way to present yourself. But if you are flexing hard, it then turns into a Figure or Body-muscle pose. Do not flex. Right arm down would look fine too.

FIGURE a-3:

This is a good example of a Bikini stance, pose. Often used in the lineup and during your individual presentation. How you shift and place your weight, hold in your stomach, hold up your head and back, will determine how well you score, so you have to nail this pose. Lots of practice.

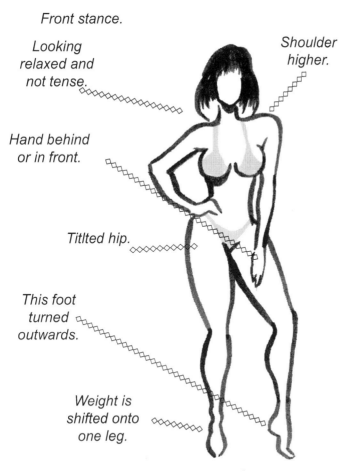

Front stance.

Looking relaxed and not tense.

Shoulder higher.

Hand behind or in front.

Titlted hip.

This foot turned outwards.

Weight is shifted onto one leg.

FIGURE a-3-b

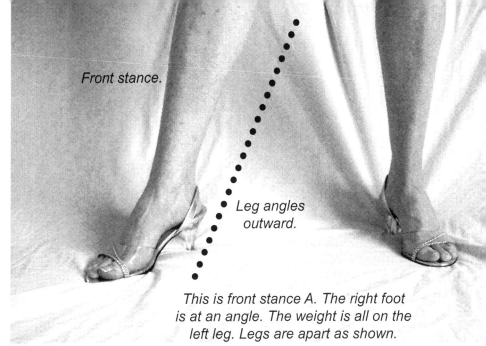

Front stance.

Leg angles outward.

This is front stance A. The right foot is at an angle. The weight is all on the left leg. Legs are apart as shown.

FIGURE a-4

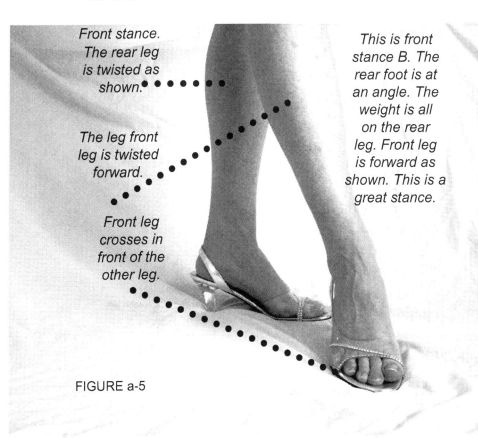

Front stance. The rear leg is twisted as shown.

This is front stance B. The rear foot is at an angle. The weight is all on the rear leg. Front leg is forward as shown. This is a great stance.

The leg front leg is twisted forward.

Front leg crosses in front of the other leg.

FIGURE a-5

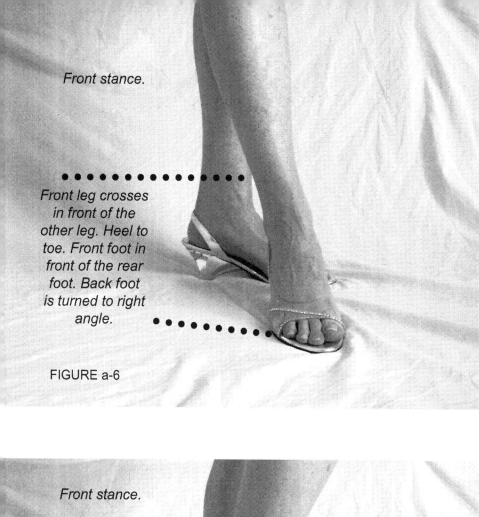

Front stance.

Front leg crosses in front of the other leg. Heel to toe. Front foot in front of the rear foot. Back foot is turned to right angle.

FIGURE a-6

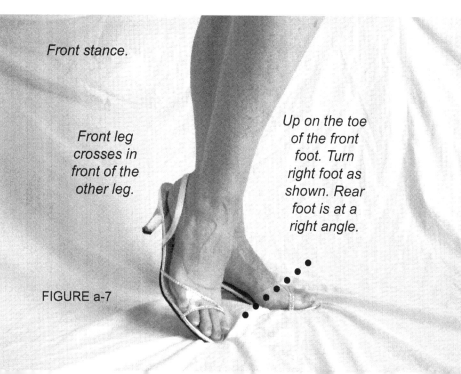

Front stance.

Front leg crosses in front of the other leg.

Up on the toe of the front foot. Turn right foot as shown. Rear foot is at a right angle.

FIGURE a-7

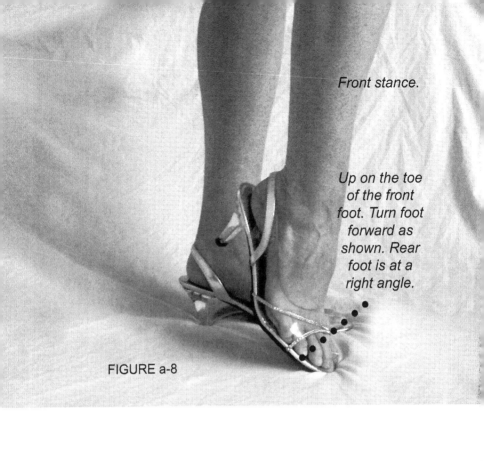

Front stance.

Up on the toe of the front foot. Turn foot forward as shown. Rear foot is at a right angle.

FIGURE a-8

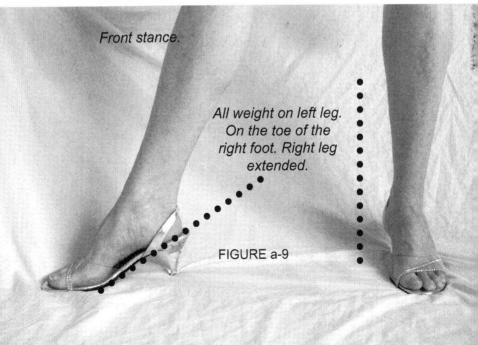

Front stance.

All weight on left leg. On the toe of the right foot. Right leg extended.

FIGURE a-9

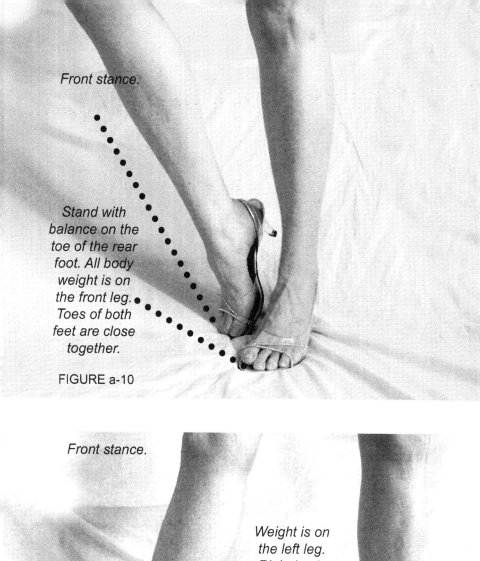

Front stance.

Stand with balance on the toe of the rear foot. All body weight is on the front leg. Toes of both feet are close together.

FIGURE a-10

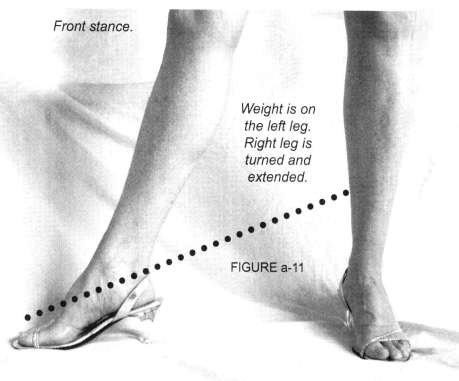

Front stance.

Weight is on the left leg. Right leg is turned and extended.

FIGURE a-11

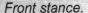

Front stance.

Feet close and turned in. This can actually look great, but can appear awkward. If you have the structure for this pose you can get away with it. Both hands are on both hips, knees are turned in slightly.

Front foot forward with 10% tilt inward.. Weight on rear leg. Rear leg forward. Front leg ever so slightly turned inward.

FIGURE a-12

Front stance.

Weight is on both legs but mainly on the left leg.

FIGURE a-13

Heels together. Feet at 90 degree angles as shown.

Foot turned as shown.

Rear stance.

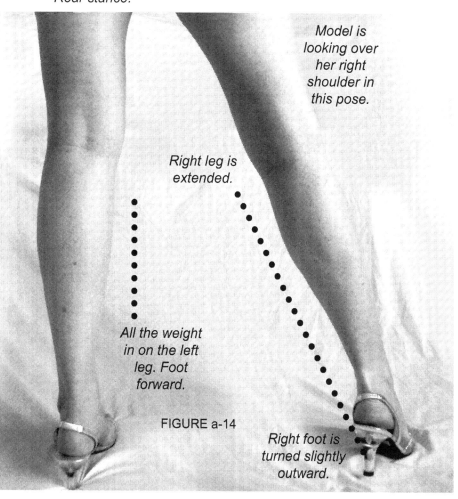

Model is
looking over
her right
shoulder in
this pose.

Right leg is
extended.

All the weight
in on the left
leg. Foot
forward.

FIGURE a-14

Right foot is
turned slightly
outward.

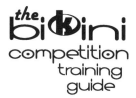

the
biⒷini
competition
training
guide

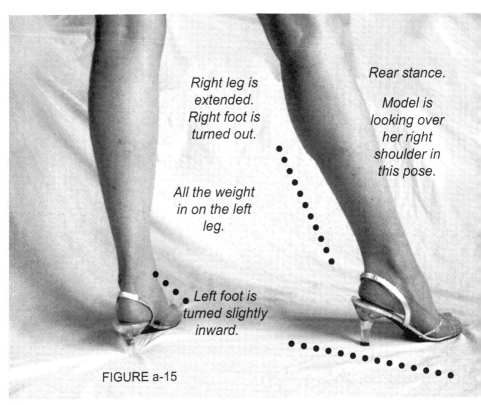

Right leg is extended. Right foot is turned out.

Rear stance.

Model is looking over her right shoulder in this pose.

All the weight in on the left leg.

Left foot is turned slightly inward.

FIGURE a-15

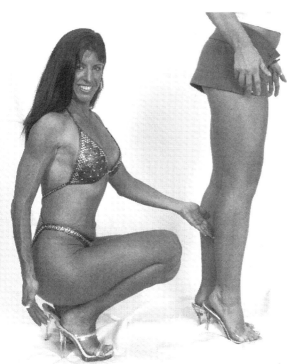

Advice from Wendy: Find someone you trust to help you practice your posing. How you walk and stand and present yourself is the fun of the show. The more you practice and feel comfortable the more fun you will have!

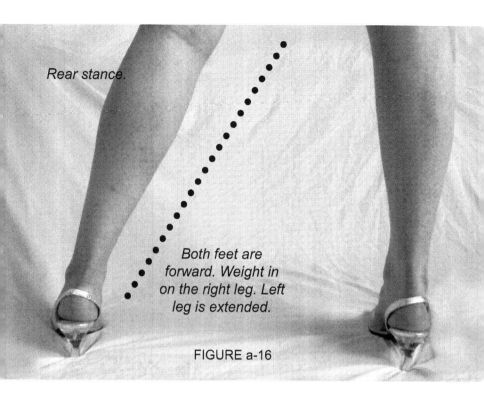

Rear stance.

Both feet are forward. Weight in on the right leg. Left leg is extended.

FIGURE a-16

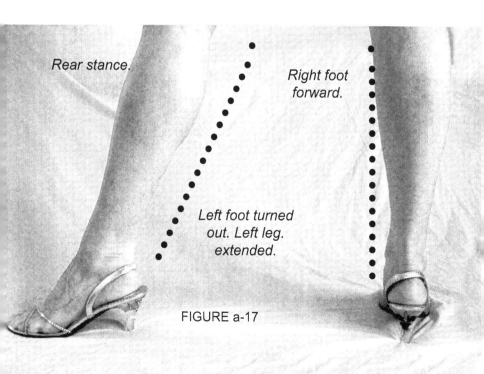

Rear stance.

Right foot forward.

Left foot turned out. Left leg. extended.

FIGURE a-17

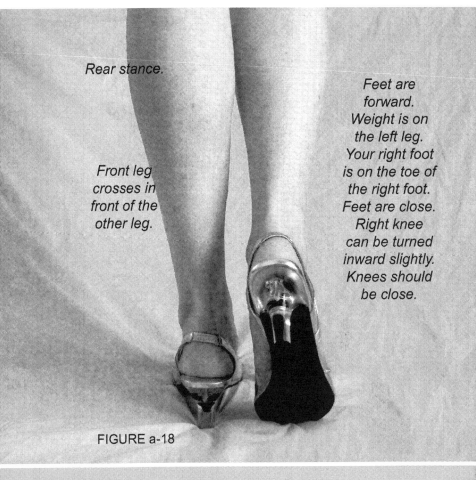

Rear stance.

Feet are forward. Weight is on the left leg. Your right foot is on the toe of the right foot. Feet are close. Right knee can be turned inward slightly. Knees should be close.

Front leg crosses in front of the other leg.

FIGURE a-18

21. Foot stances to avoid:

All too often I see contests where people are just winging it. It's obvious they gave little or no thought to their presentation. And they look sort of out of place next to someone polished and poised. Standing incorrectly can ruin all your hard work. Standing wrong can make you look fat or awkward. Here are a handful of common mistakes you want to avoid when you are on stage.

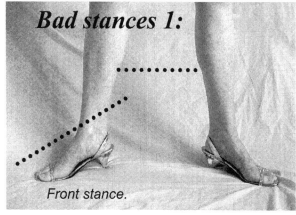

Bad stances 1:

Never pose like this please!

Feet and legs apart with weight on both legs.

FIGURE a-19

Front stance.

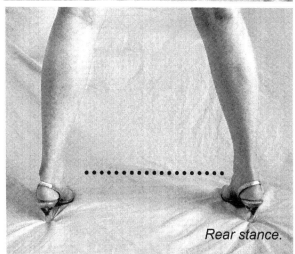

Legs apart. With feet forward, outward or inward as shown. Never pose like this!

FIGURE a-20

Rear stance.

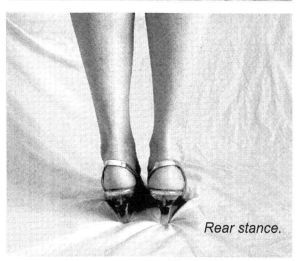

Legs locked or bent and heels together. Do not do this!

FIGURE a-21

Rear stance.

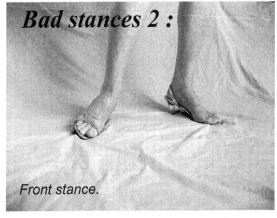

Bad stances 2 :

Front stance.

Standing normally as if waiting in the grocery line.

Right leg extended on the side of the right foot.

FIGURE a-22

Never pose like this please!

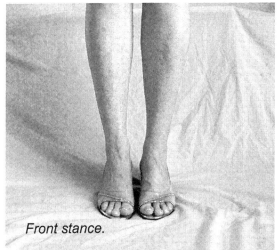

Front stance.

Feet forward and together.

FIGURE a-23

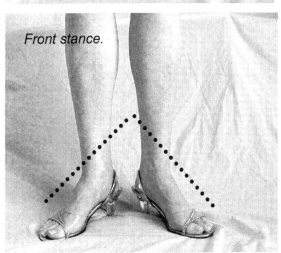

Front stance.

Never pose like this please!

Heels together and feet turned outward.

FIGURE a-24

22. The Prejudging:

Posing:
You may find yourself on stage for minutes or hours depending on how many girls are in the show. Learn to not fidget, not look bored, or stand in an unattractive manner while on stage. Always look like a super model while on stage. Here is how it goes.

Morning Prejudging:
This is where you are compared alone and then directly against the other athletes in your class.

Presentation in Bikini:

1. You walk to the center stage.

2. You stop and show yourself from the front.

3. You turn and show yourself from the side, optional.

4. Turn slowly.

5. Stop and pose, stand showing your backside.

6. Turn slowly.

7. Front pose again

8. Smile and wave and turn.

9. Walk to the side of the stage floor and stand while the other competitors present themselves.

10. Wait till everyone has presented themselves.

11. With the group return to the center of the stage and line up.

12. As a group do the front pose stance.

13. Turn as a group to the rear and stop.

14. Stand to the rear.

15. Turn back to the front and stand. Hold this pose.

16. Change positions in line, then compared again.

17. Walk offstage as a group.

STAY COOL:

No matter what happens stay calm and show good sportsmanship. I have seen 6 foot girls in the short class and along with the competitors wondering what the hell is going on. Follow the judges instructions and stay cool. Everything is a learning experience. Learning to lose gracefully is as important as any lesson you might learn. Or competing in a situation that is less than perfect.

Do your best when you prepare for your show. But once you arrive at the show, have fun. Don't take it so seriously it makes you STOP HAVING FUN. It's all about being healthy and fit. If you come in dead last but still look great, you are a winner. Always keep smiling. If you do get upset, contain yourself till long after the show is over. Do not get angry in public. Hide your emotions.

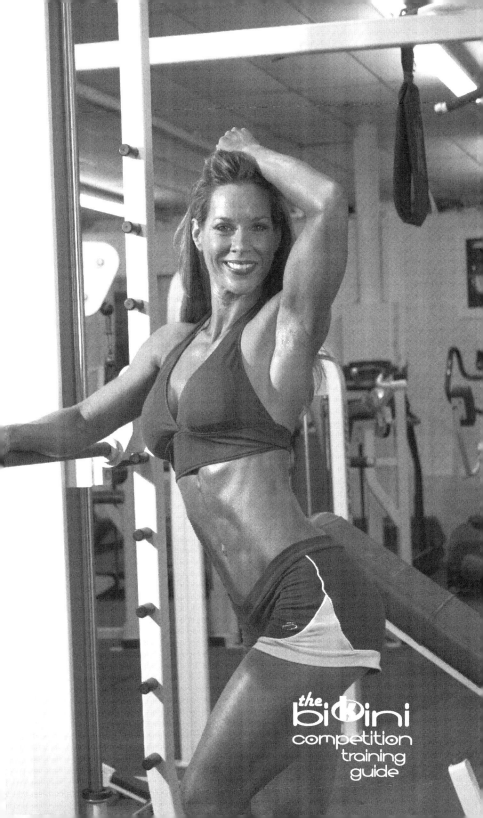

the bikini competition training guide

Individual Presentation Breakdown:

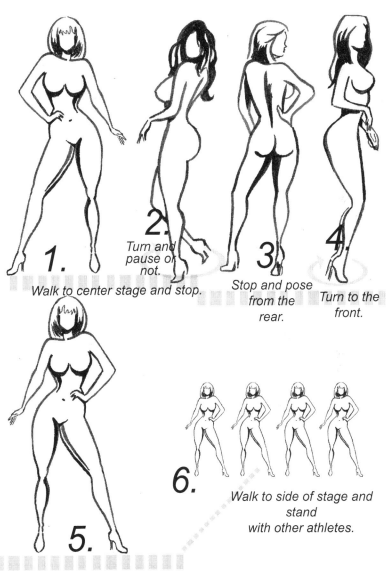

1. Walk to center stage and stop.

2. Turn and pause or not.

3. Stop and pose from the rear.

4. Turn to the front.

5. Stop and front pose.

6. Walk to side of stage and stand with other athletes.

23. The Finals:

POSING:

The evening show is a super fun time. The audience is there to see you and it is exciting. You can wear extra jewelry at night, different hair style and or bathing suit than in the morning pre-judging. You will come out and present yourself and collect your rewards. Here is what you can expect.

Evening Finals:

This is where awards are presented to the top athletes in each class.

Presentation in Bikini:

1. You walk to the center stage.

2. You stop and show yourself from the front.

3. You turn and show yourself from the side, optional.

4. Turn slowly.

5. Stop and pose, stand showing your backside.

6. Turn slowly.

7. Front pose again

8. Smile and wave and turn.

9. Walk to the side of the stage floor and stand while other athletes present themselves.

10. Wait till everyone has presented themselves.

11. With the group return to the center stage and line up.

12. Walk off stage.

13. The top people in each group are asked to return to center stage.

14. Awards are presented.

15. Photos are taken as athletes stand in the line of the top 3.

16. Walk offstage.

17. First place winner returns to compete for overall title.

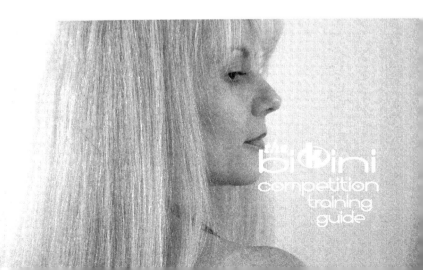

24. What to pack in your bag:

1. Your bathing suits in large freezer bags. Keep them dry and clean.

2. Warm up suit.

3. Towels, wipes and water.

4. Make-up, small scissors, false eye lashes, brush, comb.

5. Money, cell phone, phone list.

6. Driver's license, proof of payment to contest. Receipts. Application for contest and a one page typed personal biography.

7. Pam cooking spray.

8. Disposable gloves.

9. Shoes.

10. Business cards.

11. Bobby pins, safety pins.

12. Water and food.

13. Body sparkle.

14. Food and water.

15. Clothes to change into later.

16. Jewelry for the show.

17. Pen and address book.

18. Feminine products.

19. Always place your contest number or button in your bag in a plastic bag. Do not lose your number.

20. Bikini Bite: Glue to stick that suit to your body.

21. Instant tanning products.

22. Curling irons, hair spray, mirror.

23. Toothbrush, paste, floss and gum.

24. Address of contest venue. Map to the contest. Phone number of contest.

25. Camera. Extra suit and shoes.

26. Someone to help you keep track of all your stuff while you compete. (They may not fit in the bag and should not be left unattended backstage).

25. 10 days out from your contest:

This is not the time for experimentation or doing anything radical. No last minute fat loss programs or starving or anything like that. You should be fit, tan and ready to go. The last 10 days is about not making any mistakes that could **derail your plan of success.** Do not lose or try to lose weight before the show. Your suit may not fit correctly. Your body should already be there.

What we do want you to do, is to come into the show the best you can be. And that means timing the contest so you are not bloated. Sometimes a woman can hold water before her period. It's best to avoid competing at this time.

To go into the show your best let us take a look at the things to consider the last 10 days before your show.

CONTEST COUNT DOWN.

COUNT DOWN.	FINAL WEEK.
• • • • • • • • • • • • • •	• • • • • • • • • • •
DAY 1 DAY 2 DAY 3	DAY 4 DAY 5 DAY 6 DAY 7

Keep tanning 30 minutes a day. Do not become sunburned.

Stop eating protein shakes 10 days out. Stick with fish, and small amounts of chicken and beef.

Eat small meals 5 times a day.

Avoid sugars and alcohol.

Nap extra and sleep 8 hours a night.

Eat slightly less food overall at each meal.

Eat high protein for 4 days (days 7 to day 3 counting down) and then switch to high carbs for the last 2 days before the show.

The day before the show: Dehydrate the day before the show. This flattens the abs. Do not drink all day and night and eat a small amount of carbs every 2 or 3 hours. Consult with a Doctor (MD) as dehydration is dangerous. And yes, it works very well.

FINAL 3 days.

COMPETITION DAY.

DAY 8   DAY 9   DAY 10   **DAY 11**

Drink extra water all week before the day before the show.

Stop all exercise about 4 days out from the show and reduce calories accordingly.

Take a bowel cleanser or water loss pill of some sort 24 to 48 hours before the show.

Stay off your feet. Literally the day before the show. Rest your legs.

Eat a small high carb meal the morning of the show like pancakes and syrup. Load up on energy. Drink very little water the morning of the show.

Eat a small high calorie meal the day of the show. Drink 6 to 8 oz. of water at lunch and dinner.

Cut out salt 3 days before the show.

Do not tan the last 2 days before the show.

Moisturize your skin 3x a day or more for one week minimum. Avoid dry skin.

If changing the diet is a problem (carbs and proteins and all that) do this instead:

Eat normally the last 10 days. Cut out salt the last 3 days. Do not over-eat.

Eat slightly less food the last 10 days avoiding meat and protein shakes the last 5 days.

Do not eat after 6 in the evening.

Avoid sugars, and high calory liquids.

On days 2 and 1, eat high carbs and little protein. Drink extra water on day 2 and none on day 1 (counting down, day 1 is the day before the contest).

On day 1 do not drink any water and eat lightly all day.

Wear a warm up suit and heat up your body and break a deep sweat for 30 minutes.

You can also do this the morning of the show to shed more water.

Eat lightly the day before the show. No heavy meals.

Rest well for 24 to 36 hours before the show.

Ice your face the evening and morning of the show to reduce face swelling.

Apply preparation H, or other skin tightening lotions to the skin to loose skin areas, the morning of the show, under eyes and so on.

PROGRESS CHART

Nothing is more motivating than success. It feeds upon itself. It's important to keep track of your measurements so you can see your progress. Measure once every 2 weeks to stay motivated.

Measurement	Week 0	Week 2	Week 4	Week 6	Week 8	Week 10
Weight						
Waist						
Hips						
Neck						

TOTAL LOST INCHES:

WHAT TO EXPECT

WEEKS 1-2

Weight loss will be dramatic for some as the healthy foods impact the body. Up to 12 pounds!

WEEKS 5-7

Weight loss is steady now. Your body is primed to drop even more fat. Start your double cardio.

WEEKS 3-4

You will feel better everyday now. The body thrives on the exercise and good food. Another 5 to 10 pounds lost.

WEEKS 8-10

Depending on your starting point, you may even see your abs now. Up to 30 pounds gone!

Measurement	Week 12	Week 14	Week 16	Week 18	Week 20	Week 22
Weight						
Waist						
Hips						
Neck						

TOTAL LOST INCHES:

Measurement	Week 24	Week 26	Week 28	Week 30	Week 32	Week 34
Weight						
Waist						
Hips						
Neck						

TOTAL LOST INCHES:

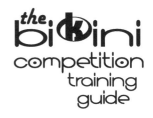

26. The rules of exercise:

1. Consult with a doctor to make sure you are healthy enough to work out and exercise.

2. Break into training or new exercises slowly. Never train to a point that it makes you sore.

3. Warm up and cool down every time you train. 5 to 10 minutes.

4. Never train to exhaustion or over-tiredness.

5. Never do exercises that hurt.

6. Resistance train 2x a week.

7. Always rest several days between resistance workouts in order for your body to recover.

8. Perform 2 to 3 sets of all exercises. The first set is a warm-up set. The second or third set is a high intensity set. On these sets, work really hard.

9. Perform anywhere from 10 to 20 repetitions on each set.

10. Train the body head to toe. Train legs, torso, and arms every time you do resistance training.

11. Stretch after training to maintain flexibility. Yoga, stretching, and swimming can help you stay flexible.

12. Practice balancing exercises for several minutes each day. Tai-Chi or Yoga is great for this.

13. Practice breathing exercises for several minutes everyday.

14. Aerobic or cardio exercise is done for 30 to 60 minutes 5x a week. Double cardio sessions can be done each day. One session in the morning and one in the late afternoon is ideal.

15. Every time you train, try to slightly increase the intensity of your training. Make your increases small so you don't get hurt or overly sore. You can increase workout intensity by doing one of the following: adding reps to each set, adding sets, performing new exercises, switching from machines to free weights or bands, increasing resistance, or increasing distance, effort or time. This is called exercising progressively.

27. Sculpting the Bikini winning body.

The Look of a Bikini winner.

Champions are made not born. But there are people that have great bodies and don't have to work hard for them. Others have to put in the time to craft a champion body. I have seen women of 200 pounds diet down to 105 and look crazy sexy with a perfect body. You never know what you have till you get all the fat off and take a look.

The Bikini champion look is not about looking like a bodybuilder. In fact that is not the look you want. You don't want to have developed upper body muscle mass and large legs as a Bikini competitor. If you are disposed to being muscular you should think about Figure competition or bodybuilding. Bikini is not about muscle or looking muscular.

Focus on the right stuff.

You want a feminine hour glass figure with a small waist and round tight hip and buttock area. Also your legs should be fat free but not too muscular. So what is the look besides slim and fat free? The look is not manly, the opposite of that, more like a ballroom dancer than a runner or weight trainer look. The back and arms are NOT muscular. The legs are not overly ripped or large.

The Bikini champion can be full figured, being thin is not the look, but she has to look balanced and feminine. Large ripped muscles are not feminine in the Bikini sense.

So **avoid** accentuating areas (like arms or back) that don't need to be built up at all.

A firm, flat, midsection is the next essential part of your winning look. You can't have flabby abdominals and compete to win.

Many champions do not train their upper body at all except with light weights and training abs. Training light for your upper body is a good idea to avoid becoming too muscular. If you are very thin, adding some meat to your upper body will help you look better. Too thin is not a winning look. A full, fat free look, is the winning look. When I mean full, I mean, the muscle on the athlete does not look "hard" or "shredded" or overly defined. It's not a muscle contest.

Continued 7 pages over.

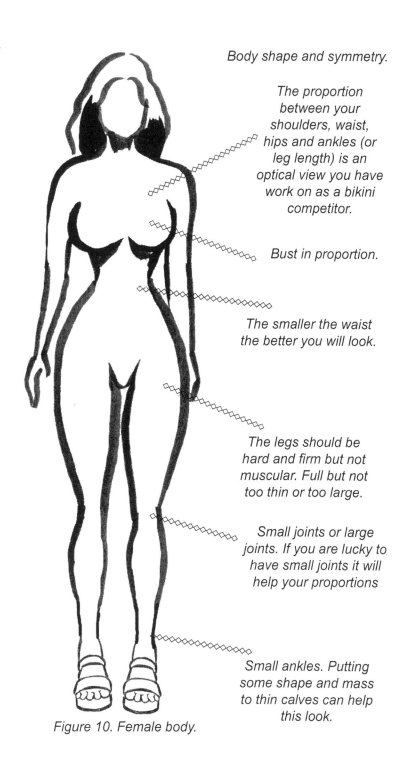

Body shape and symmetry.

The proportion between your shoulders, waist, hips and ankles (or leg length) is an optical view you have work on as a bikini competitor.

Bust in proportion.

The smaller the waist the better you will look.

The legs should be hard and firm but not muscular. Full but not too thin or too large.

Small joints or large joints. If you are lucky to have small joints it will help your proportions

Small ankles. Putting some shape and mass to thin calves can help this look.

Figure 10. Female body.

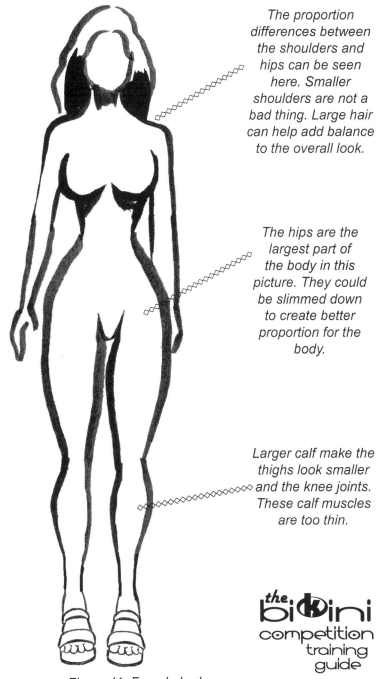

The proportion differences between the shoulders and hips can be seen here. Smaller shoulders are not a bad thing. Large hair can help add balance to the overall look.

The hips are the largest part of the body in this picture. They could be slimmed down to create better proportion for the body.

Larger calf make the thighs look smaller and the knee joints. These calf muscles are too thin.

the
bi**k**ini
competition
training
guide

Figure 11. Female body.

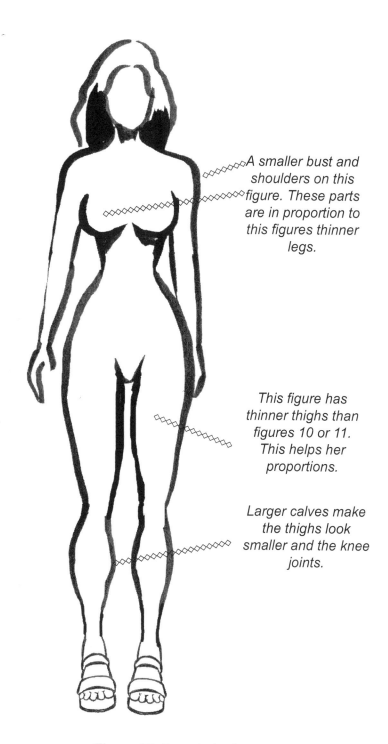

A smaller bust and shoulders on this figure. These parts are in proportion to this figures thinner legs.

This figure has thinner thighs than figures 10 or 11. This helps her proportions.

Larger calves make the thighs look smaller and the knee joints.

Figure 12. Female body.

28. Body shaping tips for abs:

1. Do stomach vacuums and high rep abdominal exercises for abs.

2. Do twisting movements for abs. Rotation of the upper torso.

3. Never use weight on your abs.

4. Never over-eat or distend or stretch the stomach.

5. Don't get pregnant more than once every 5 years.

6. Hold the abs in mentally throughout the day.

7. Do abs for 5 minutes 3x a day or more.

8. Train abs on an empty stomach.

9. Only train abs 6 weeks before a show. Do not train them too much. Avoid thickening the stomach muscle wall.

10. No dead lifts or squats with heavy breathing.

29. Body shaping tips, legs:

1. If squats or weight training causes your legs to become too muscular (you may already have enough muscle mass on your legs) avoid this type of exercise.

2. Perform high reps for leg exercises.

3. Focus on butt training more than thigh training.

4. If you have legs with short thighs or stocky thighs do forward kicks to make the leg muscles develop from the crotch to the knee. This gives a long leg look to your thighs.

5. If your upper thighs are too large do lots of walking and aerobic training. When squatting use light weights and focus on the bottom (not the top) of the squat movement.

6. Running can make legs look too wiry, thin or hard looking.

7. Dancing (Ballet and other forms) can add great tone to legs without building size or unsymmetrical muscle mass.

8. Stretching the leg muscles after training to give them a long smooth look.

9. Doing pilates or other forms of static holding exercises. Building tone without adding mass.

10. To add thigh mass and make a rounder butt area do squats with a wide stance. Once the body fills out, discontinue squats.

11. Swimming with a kick board to focus on legs can build beautiful legs from top to bottom.

12. To get thinner or decrease thigh mass. Choose exercises like swimming or walking that do a high volume of reps on your legs.

13. Train calves to balance the thighs.

Continued from 7 pages before.

Focusing your training time:

A tight round butt on a pair of firm smooth legs is where you want to focus your time when it comes to training. Second to focus on is abdominal. How you shape these key areas will create the foundation of your winning Bikini body. Let's focus on that look in detail.

Legs:

You don't want weight lifter's legs so building muscle with squats and leg presses MAY NOT WORK for you. Why? Because your legs develop (over time) with a manly look (muscle is heavy over the knee and outer quads, and or buttocks are too thick). So body weight squats with light dumbbells (using higher reps, 15 to 30 reps per set) and **avoiding** heavy weights **is the plan.**

Lunges with light dumbbells, leg kick-backs and ball butt lifts, and other exercises that develop a "long leg" look, can develop the legs without giving them that "bodybuilder" look.

Squats, when done light, and lunges will benefit 99% of most female Bikini athletes. Don't be afraid to do these valuable exercises.

If you are overly thin, or have a "flat butt"

syndrome, squats can and will actually develop a round buttock area and fuller, better looking thighs. Thin people who need to gain weight in order to have a more pleasing shape can benefit from squats and other leg exercises with "heavier" weights. This helps them "fill in" areas that need a fuller look.

 The idea is to stay feminine looking. Don't develop muscles that detract from that look (like back, arms and a thick waist). Also stretching, and pilates and or swimming can develop a feminine body with strong hard muscles that appear smooth without the bulky "look". Most women will not bulk up from weights but some will so how you train will effect how your muscles develop and look.

Will dancing, like ballroom, develop a great body? Yes, but so will many athletic activities. A dancer's body is not a guarantee of winning, but that look, long muscles that form a very pleasing and feminine looking leg-- with round firm buttocks and flat, fat free stomach-- is the look you are after.

 Much of your focus should be spent developing feminine legs and not muscular, thick legs.

 Eventually you have to find what works

best for you. I knew a girl who was naturally muscular. So she never trained with weights. She did lots of walking and some ab work and ate very clean. She focused on weight loss and getting thin. I have to say, she looked great.

For her, weight training, or heavy training, were counterproductive to her goal of looking slim and sexy. Over time she did return to leg training to keep her butt hard and round, but for the most part all she did was walk. And she looked great.

Big arms or a different look is not the Bikini look. How you get there will be determined by the genetic cards you were dealt. You need to figure out what will work for you. Don't try to do it "all". Just do what YOU need to do. No more and no less.

Stomach Training (abs):

Train your stomach along with your leg training. But if you find you waist thickening from training, stop training your waist.

Instead, do not train your stomach at all and focus on shrinking your waist. (See the section on waist shrinking).

Most people however, have to train their abs at least 3 times a week in order to maintain a flat stomach. For me my abs look best from daily training. You will have to figure out what works for you. Never use weights when training your abs. Body weight or lighter only. Do high repetitions on your ab training.

Once you are fat free and your abs are flat you can avoid training abs for most of your training year. Let the toned muscles shrink (atrophy) while still dieting hard. You can take additional inches and mass off your waist with this strategy. Often fat forms on our abs and won't come off. Cardio training and clean eating will destroy (reduce) this fat, instead of endless ab training. Doing abs does not burn ab fat. That is why "fat burning" exercise is used to burn fat. It works!

Too much ab training actually thickens the waist and damages your overall "thin waist" look. Don't train abs with weights. Don't train your obliques (side abs) as this makes your waist thick. Avoid anything like heavy squats, dead lift or overeating that thickens the center of the body.

Rather strengthen the core of your body (hips, low back, abs) with exercises like swimming, weights with high repetitions, palates, and body weight only abdominal training.

Once you are fat free, and your abs are flat you can do abs 6 weeks before a contest (daily) and they will be both small (from the non work) and newly "tightened" from the 6 weeks of intense training and look amazing.

So if you are already "there" only do abs before a show and you will be perfect for your show.

This is an old trick used by bodybuilders and it works if you are already "there" and just trying to get prepared for a show.

If you are still struggling just to get it all together for the first time, ignore this advice for now. But once you are "there" come back and reread this section of the manual.

A small waist. Sexy, firm legs that are not overly muscular. A tight round hard butt. That is the look you are after. That is the look you are working for.

Some girls do have pleasing shape and mass naturally. Most have to work at it, and that is okay. Some are too thick, some are too thin. Depending on your natural shape, you will have to train accordingly.

Always train (a tiny bit at least) your upper body to have healthy level of upper body tone. You don't want to be physically weak. Just avoid using heavy weights and or becoming overly muscular. If you do start to notice excessive muscle development on a certain body part, just back off.

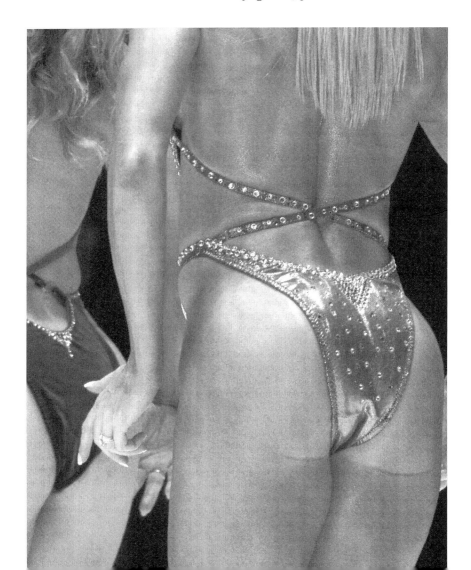

30. Leg shapes and mass:

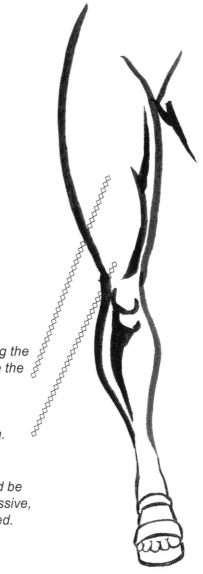

Female thigh. Avoid building the leg muscles directly above the knee and upper thigh.

Figure 15. Female thigh.

Female thigh. Legs should be shapely and toned. Not massive, large, muscular or defined.

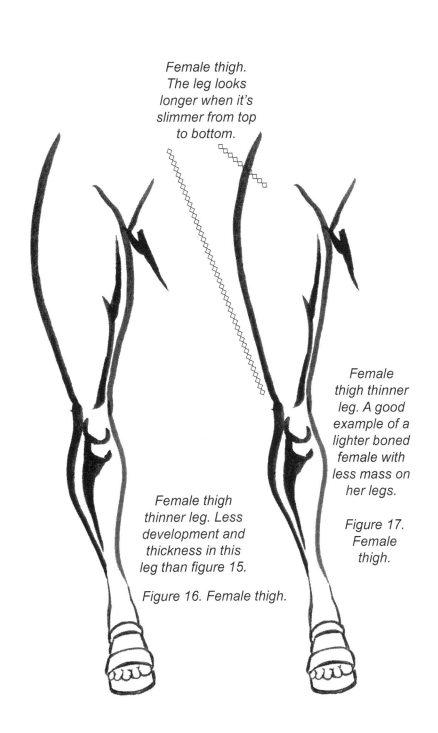

Female thigh. The leg looks longer when it's slimmer from top to bottom.

Female thigh thinner leg. A good example of a lighter boned female with less mass on her legs.

Figure 17. Female thigh.

Female thigh thinner leg. Less development and thickness in this leg than figure 15.

Figure 16. Female thigh.

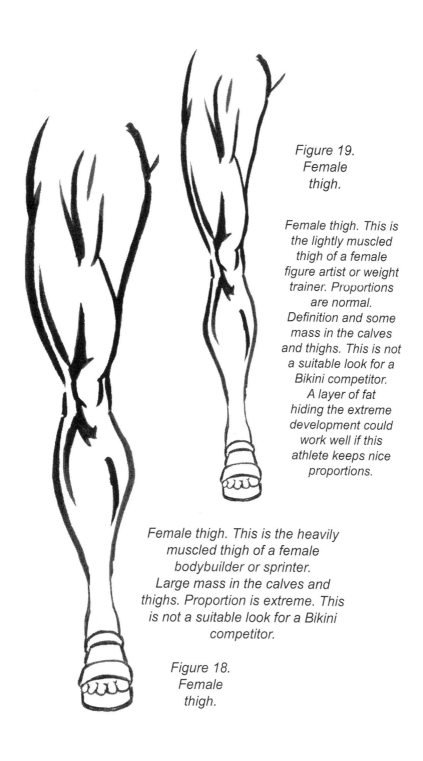

Figure 19.
Female
thigh.

Female thigh. This is
the lightly muscled
thigh of a female
figure artist or weight
trainer. Proportions
are normal.
Definition and some
mass in the calves
and thighs. This is not
a suitable look for a
Bikini competitor.
A layer of fat
hiding the extreme
development could
work well if this
athlete keeps nice
proportions.

Female thigh. This is the heavily
muscled thigh of a female
bodybuilder or sprinter.
Large mass in the calves and
thighs. Proportion is extreme. This
is not a suitable look for a Bikini
competitor.

Figure 18.
Female
thigh.

31. Buttock shapes and mass:

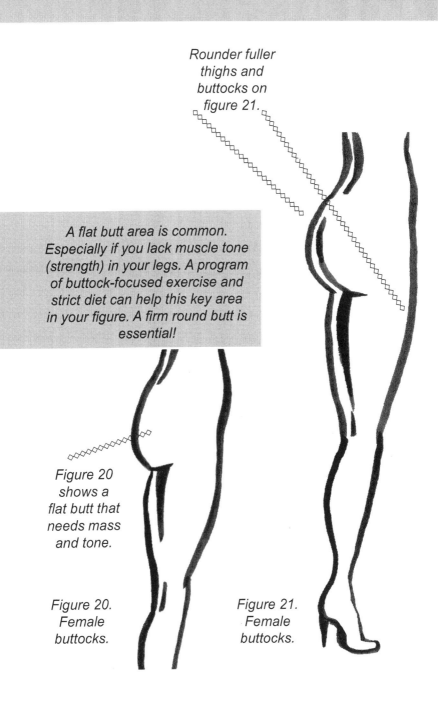

Rounder fuller
thighs and
buttocks on
figure 21.

A flat butt area is common.
Especially if you lack muscle tone
(strength) in your legs. A program
of buttock-focused exercise and
strict diet can help this key area
in your figure. A firm round butt is
essential!

Figure 20
shows a
flat butt that
needs mass
and tone.

Figure 20.
Female
buttocks.

Figure 21.
Female
buttocks.

32. Grooming. The make up and hair artist.

Competition is show business. It's theater.

Dolly Parton always looks great on her videos. The wigs, the make up, the style all adds up to a pleasing whole.

Your hair and make up can make or break you. It will help you win or it will cause your loss. My advice is, if you are not sure how to do hair and makeup, HIRE someone who is good at makeup and hair (especially for your first show or two). Have them teach you how to do your hair and makeup so you look good on stage. If you are able, hire them and have them do your makeup for you backstage or right before your show. Same with hair, or buy really good wigs. You might have a "hair expert" and a separate "make up expert" to assist you in your contest preparations.

Let me tell you how important this "grooming" business all is.

I was back stage at a show when I noticed a girl that looked like anything but a winner. Her hair, make up, and so on, were a wreck, she looked like she had slept under her car and come into the show. Her skin was dark, but looked old like a leather chair.

About 30 minutes later she walked on stage. She had glossed her tan skin with some sort of oil and now she looked pretty good. She had on a blond wig and her make up was perfect. And she walked, smiled and worked the judges and audience like a pro. Her teeth and smile were radiant. I did not know it was even the same person. Not till later did I put it all together. This person was able to go from zero to hero in 30 minutes by

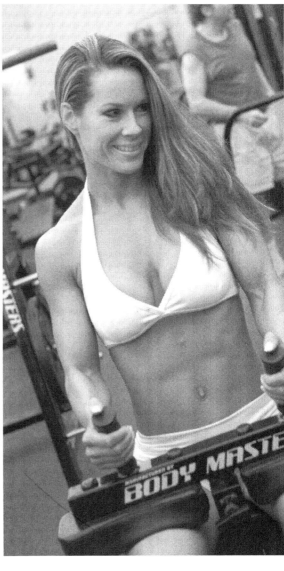

knowing how to groom to the max.

After she won the show, she came backstage, and took off her wig. "Wow that is hot!" she said, holding her trophy and the wig. Her hair was jet black and short. Unlike her long, blond flowing wig! Up close you could see the heavy face make up (looked perfect on stage) and 1 inch long eye lashes. I asked her how old she was. She said "older than you!", and I was 44 at the time! Grooming is the icing on the cake, the glossy polish on the car, the final coat of paint on your new house. Without it, the thing seems incomplete and IT IS!

You must focus on your grooming at a professional level to successfully compete

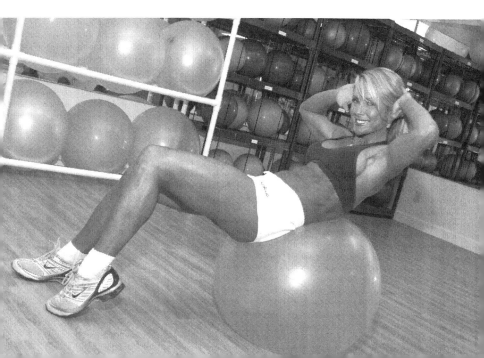

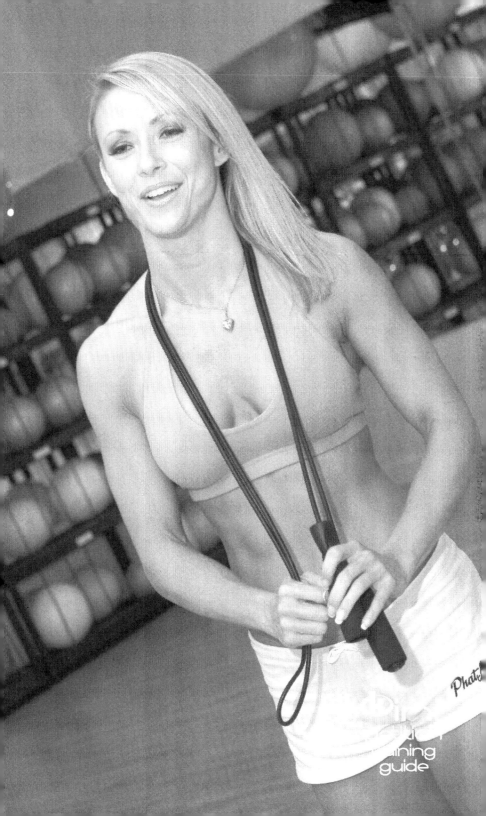

training
guide

in Bikini competition.

There is no doubt that your body is important for winning Bikini contests (you need a great figure) but so is your overall look. From your toes to your nose you should be on top of your grooming. If you are not a grooming or makeup expert you need to find someone to help you learn what you need to know.

Never compete without makeup, clean polished hair, velvet looking skin and a great smile. These are some of your most important weapons on the Bikini field of battle. Do not leave them at home or "forget" about them. You will be embarrassed in competition if you do forget them, and that won't be any fun for you.

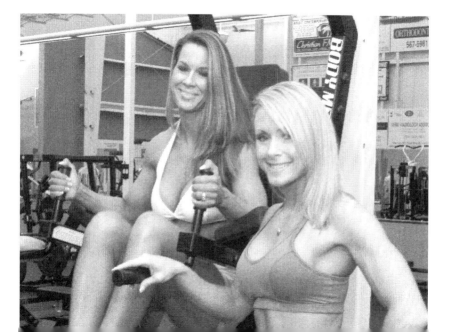

33. The shape of your head affects your look.

The outline or contour or profile line of your body is an important thing to consider. How your hair shape (mass and shape actually) effects the overall balance of your body. That is why Dolly Parton wears giant wigs to balance her giant boobs and hips. If her head was small she would like a light bulb head! Consider a wig to get your head shape perfect. Not all of us are born with perfect hair. Extensions, braids, coloring are all ideas we can use to make our hair more dynamic for competition.

Imagine this: Two girls are tied at a bikini contest with equal bodies. Guess what? The one with the better hair will win. Good hair counts.

For example, if you are super thin or slim with giant Dallas Cheerleader hair, it's going to unbalance your overall look and make your small hips and small chest look smaller! The upturned broom look!

The contour shape, the mass of your hair, should balance your body and make it more attractive. Bust and hip ratios are something all women are thinking about, then add in shoulders and hair and we have the complete package.

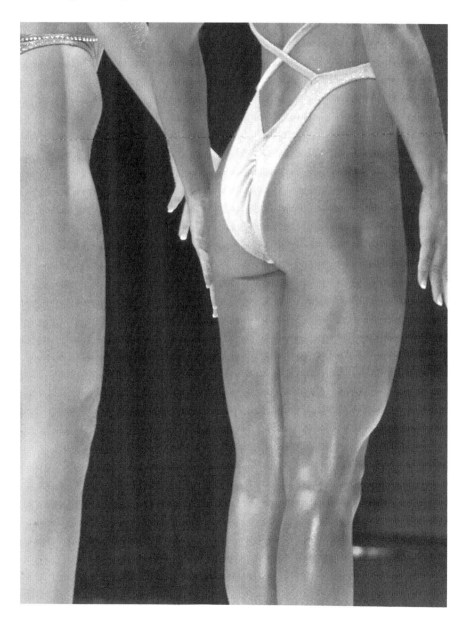

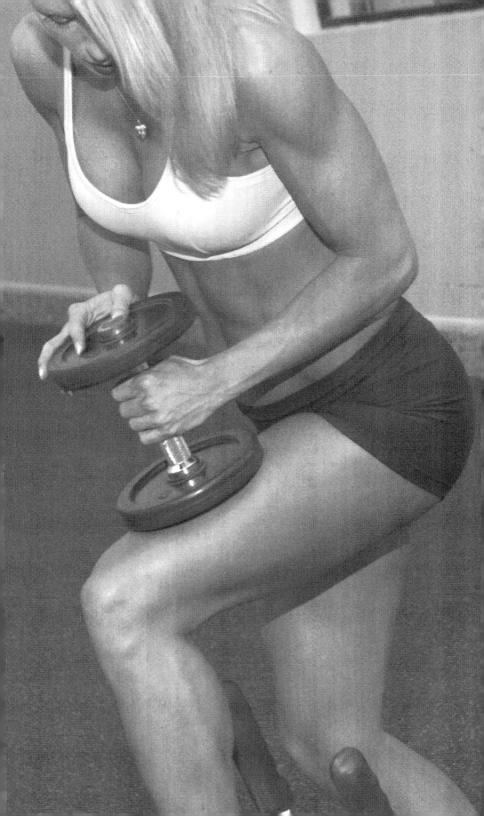

34. Skin and tanning.

You need a deep tan to compete. A tan can make or break you. You can, and should, use sunless tanning products, but they look best on top of a **real tan.**

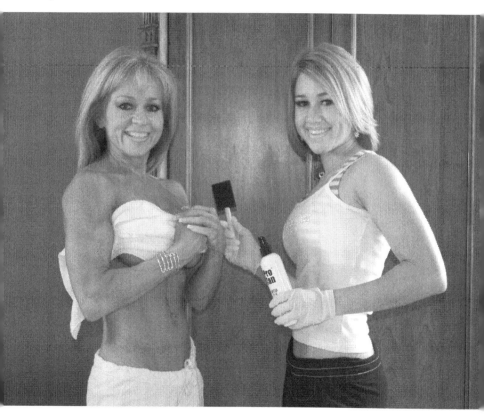

If you are serious about competing you will need a tan. A real tan. And you will need face make-up so when you compete, your face (which you should avoid tanning) is the same color as your body. Avoid having a tan body and a white face. It looks odd on stage. Your face and body should be the same color.

If possible give yourself time to get a good base tan. 3 to 4 weeks. You can use the real sun or a tanning booth. Even 10 sessions in the sun can give you enough of a real tan so that when you add on a fake tan it looks good.

Try various sunless tanning agents and see what is best for your skin type. Some look orange-colored on certain people. The orange look is one you want

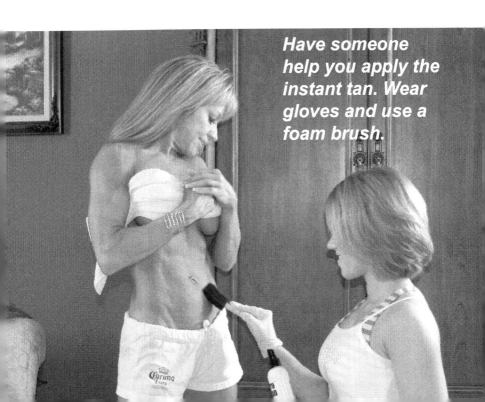

Have someone help you apply the instant tan. Wear gloves and use a foam brush.

to avoid. Apply only a small amount at first and make sure you are not allergic to the sunless tanning product. Avoid contact with nice clothing, hair, hands, feet, carpets, towels, and nice furniture. Dyes come off on everything, so be careful!

Fake tanning. From spray tanning to home products there are many "sunless tanning" products. Plan on using a product that works for you to compete with. Even if you already tan you will want to spray tan or add artificial color to your skin in order to compete and look dark on stage.

A good tan can win a contest. White untanned looking skin can lose a contest. Keep your skin moisturized and avoid becoming sunburned.

There are strategies for getting a great tan and looking as if you are tan (using sunless tanning products) that you can use to compete with. Use plastic gloves and foam brushes to apply fake tanning dyes to your skin. Put old sheets on your bed and wear old clothes to avoid staining. Have a friend help you paint your body. It's hard to paint yourself, especially your backside.

If you can't tan do not compete. You are wasting your time. I have seen more than one "loser" come back in 2 months with a

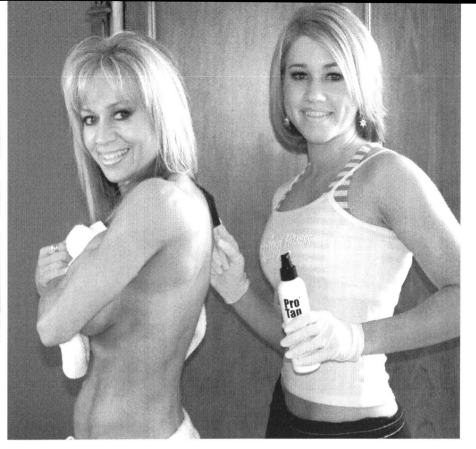

deep tan and win the entire show. Do not think you can skimp by on any part of Bikini contest preparation. Your tan is crucial to your winning.

ONE DAY TAN PLAN

This is the one day tan plan for people that have to do it all in one day.

1. Start with a good base tan.

2. Apply 1 to 2 coats of color to your skin 4 to 6 times today. Allow 2 hours to dry between coats.

3. Plan to lock yourself in a (hotel) room all day, stay naked, and tan yourself every 2 hours.

4. Morning of the show. Use an instant tanning agent like dream tan (rub on and rub off like make up) if you are still not tan enough.

5. Apply again before the evening show.

6. Avoid showering or hot showers. Cold fast showers only. Do not scrub your skin hard. The skin dye will come off in a blotchy pattern if you shower and the rub your skin. Avoid tight clothes.

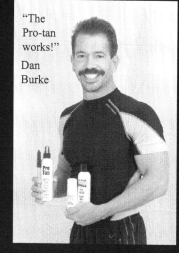

"The Pro-tan works!"

Dan Burke

THREE DAY TAN PLAN

1. Start with a good base tan.

1. Wednesday night or 3 days out from the show begin dye tanning. Two coats of dye tan Wednesday night.

2. Thursday and Friday nights, two coats of dye both nights.

3. Avoid hot water showering. Shower fast in cold water. Pat dry lightly with old towels. The skin dye will come off in a blotchy pattern if you shower and / or the dye rubs off. Avoid tight clothes. The dye will rub off at friction points like your armpits, and back of legs.

4. The 3 day tan plan works well because it gives the dye time to dry, soak into the skin between applications, smooth out blotchy spots and looks better than a one day tan application. By the third day it looks very good. This is the suggested method to tan. All the pros use it and so should you.

6. Apply an instant tanning product directly before you compete to get even darker. Dream tan or similar product.

7. Cover bruises, stretch marks or other skin marks with body make-up.

NO TAN PLAN

1. Forget to get a good base tan.

2. Apply make up or spray tan the day before the show.

3. Look pale and washed out (or maybe even orange) on stage.

4. Lose your contest.

5. The moral is: never compete without a good tan plan!

35. Choosing your suit:

The body makes the suit. But the wrong suit can lose you a contest. The wrong suit can make you look badly proportioned or awkward. The right suit should do the opposite. The right suit compliments your body. It's very important that you choose a suit that looks perfect on your body.

This may mean having a suit custom made. This is **usually a smart idea** as **nothing fits better** than clothes made by a skilled crafts person especially for you. If you have the money, have a suit made for your body. You will be glad you did.

Wait till you have

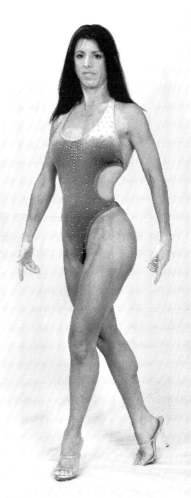

lost all your weight before you are fitted for your suit.

Can you get away with a store suit? Of course! It's up to you to decide.

Always trim off the excess strings from your suit so they are not dangling all over the place. Once you tie the suit in place, cut off the extra string with a sharp scissors.

You can have a top made with padding or even a water bra or silicone bra sewn into the bathing suit top. Or you can wear a bra or add in breast forms, under the suit top. This can add volume and shape to your breasts. Consider wearing some sort of shaping bra or top when you compete even if you have "perfect" breasts already.

Avoid white or light colors. They get dirty very easily from tanning dyes.

There are many styles of suits. Some with sequins and even lights. Choose a suit that fits well and covers your body in all the right places. A suit too small is as bad as one too big. It looks wrong on the athlete.

Styles of suits change from region to region and it's not often clear what is best. Here are some rules to help you choose a good suit.

Avoid a super weird design that looks more like a stripper outfit or costume. Stick with traditional suit cuts and you will always look good.

Solid colors and or darker colors work best. Hawaiian prints, fur suits, leather, or other odd ball choices can be distracting for the judges. Stick with solid colors, even if it's gold sparkle cloth. Small chains, jewelry, rhinestones, or other things on the suit are fine as long as they look good. Don't look like a show girl. No feathers or weird stuff.

Some contests make you wear their standard suit. One stock suit for all the competitors. If this happens to you, good luck. Often wearing a shaping bra, a smoothing girdle (spanks) under a suit like this can be very helpful. If you have to wear a stock suit be sure to use body glue like Bikini Bite and stick it (the suit) to your body so it does not move all over the place.

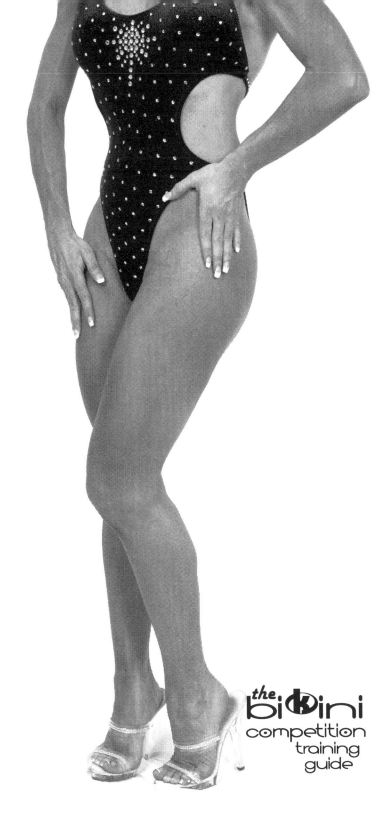

the bikini
competition
training
guide

36. Exercise and Split Routines:

Why exercise? To shape, firm, tone and strengthen our bodies. To look awesome.

What can it do for you? If your legs are thin, fill them in by training legs with weight exercises like squats and lunges. If your butt is flat, you can make it round by doing squats and lunges (just to name two of hundreds of possible butt rounding exercises). If you have no ab muscles, you can make some by training your abdominals. Flabby arms? You can firm them up fast with weight training. It's a fact. So some of your time should be spent doing weight training to firm up and shape the muscles on your body.

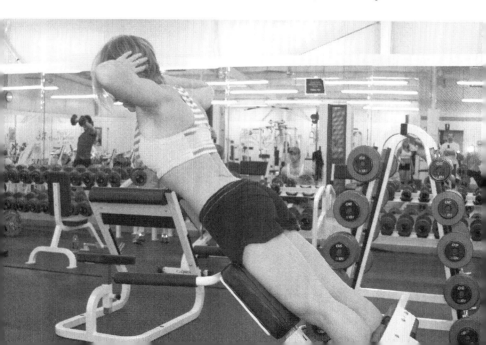

You need to divide your training time into two parts: training for fat loss doing fat burning exercise (we call this cardio) and muscle firming exercise (resistance training like weight training). You have to make time to do both.

Most people find that breaking their workout into training days (training legs on Monday and arms

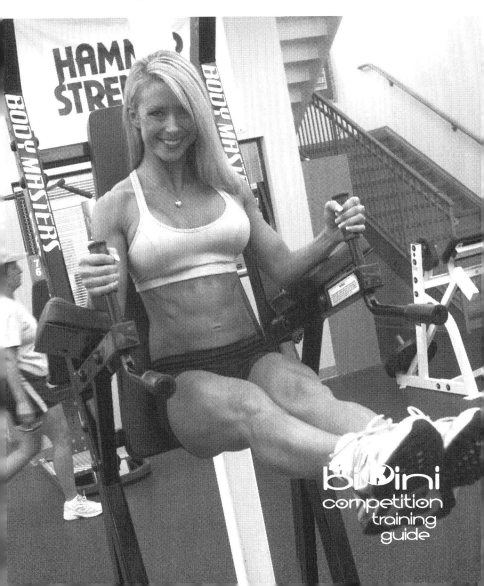

bikini
competition
training
guide

on Tuesday and so on) is a prudent way to approach their training program. It's up to you to decide if and when you want to split your training. It's not mandatory that you do so to make progress, but most people, adopt some sort of a training split program. Even if it is simply weights one day and cardio the next day.

You do not need hard ripped muscles to be a bikini champion. You need to be toned. Your flesh needs a healthy firm look, but not that of a man with muscles. What is tone? Low level muscularity?

Firmness of flesh is created by muscle. When you get stronger and or exercise you send electrical impulses through your muscles and proteins bind together. If you are fat free and your skin is very thin, you can see the muscles under the skin. You do not need to "see" muscles to be a bikini athlete. What you need is tone. Lots of electrical impulses traveling through your muscles so it looks firm. You can have a layer of fat both on your skin and inside the muscle (interstitial fat) and still look and be very firm. In women this small amount of fat tends to look good. About 10 to 12% body fat on a fit, toned woman looks very good.

You do not need to lose all your fat to be a

bikini athlete. Looking super hard or muscular is not at all the look you are after.

You want to modify and create a routine and diet

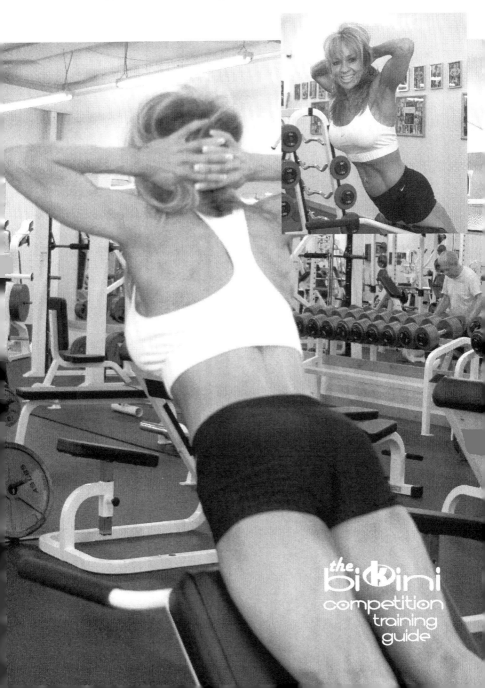

plan that works for you. Stick with the basics and you can go a long way.

Most bikini athletes train daily either doing cardio training or resistance training. Some days you end up doing both. How you divide up your training will depend upon your goals, motivation, and time available. Most people feel that if they had more time they could

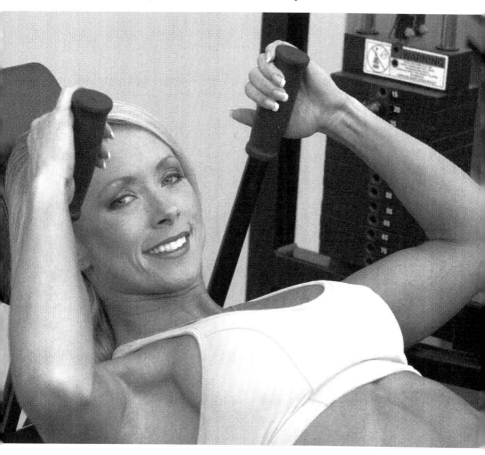

make better progress. This is not really true. Two or three hours of exercise a week is more than enough time to form a fantastic body.

Training hours each day does not yield faster or better results. A simple exercise routine for 1 to 3 hours a week can give you about 100% of what you need to be a champion! Don't let the myth of limited time slow you down.

How should you go about breaking up your training? What is best?

A simple routine can work well. Just by choosing about ten exercises and doing 3 to 4 sets twice per week, can have a profound effect on how you look and feel. The key to exercise is not frequency or duration but how hard you work. 30 minutes of

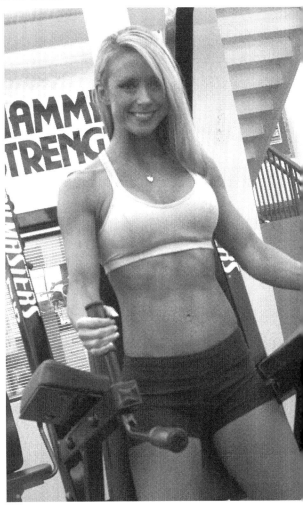

hard training is better than hours fooling around. When you train, even if it is only for 10 minutes, do your best to give yourself a good workout. Always try to do a little more or work a little bit harder, each time you train. You do not need a complicated training plan to make progress. You do not need exotic equipment. What you need is effort. Desire. You have to learn to safely push yourself every time you train. Never train to exhaustion, but feel free to train hard. Break a sweat. Breath hard. It's good for you. A short routine done once or twice a week can make you stronger and more fit and shape your body.

We suggest a full body workout after you've built up to it, because it works. How hard you work is the determining factor of success, not how often you train (up to a point) or what kind of equipment you use. Split training offers no "magic". In fact it's easier to overtrain on a split program. And easier to stay weak and think you are training. Before you do a split workout or start adding in exercises to your routine, get strong on the basic movements and then move on.

Split routines also mean training different muscle groups on different days.

There are several ways to split your workouts. You have to decide what muscle groups to combine, how to incorporate rest days, and so on.

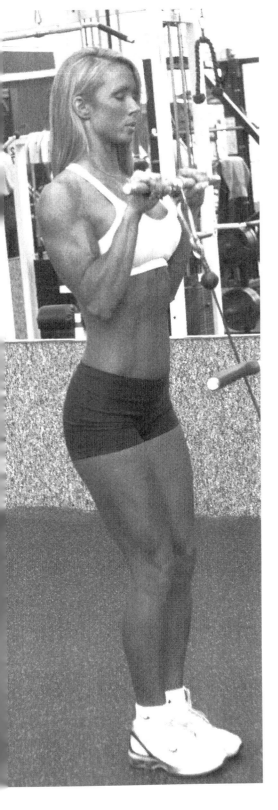

We present full body routines. As a bikini athlete you may find that it's too much upper body work. If so, then spend your time on other things. As mentioned, focus on your legs, abdominals and buttocks. These are your key areas of focus as a bikini athlete.

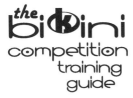

Training Program 1:

Resistance Training with weights:

30 minutes of resistance training. Work out two times per week. Perform 6 exercises that train the entire body. 1 to 3 sets of each exercise, 15 to 20 repetitions per set.

EXERCISE LIST:

Ball ab sit ups.
Leg pullups on the floor.
Ball butt lifts 2 legs.
Dumbbell (DB) squats.
DB one arm rows.
DB chest press on flat bench.

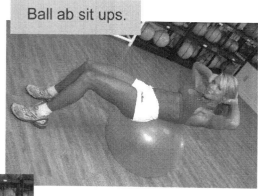

Ball ab sit ups.

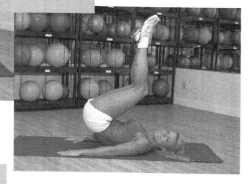

Leg pullups on the floor.

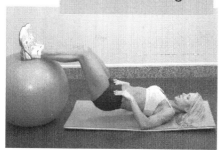

Ball butt lift 2 legs.

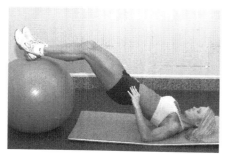

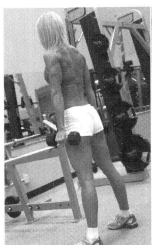

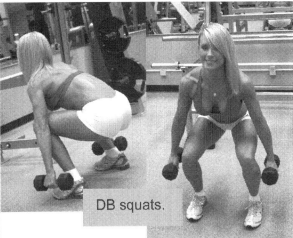

DB squats.

DB one arm rows.

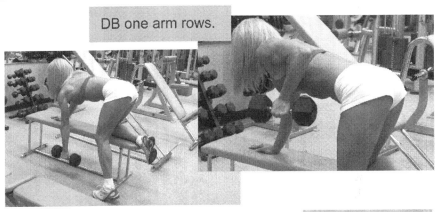

DB chest press
on a flat bench.

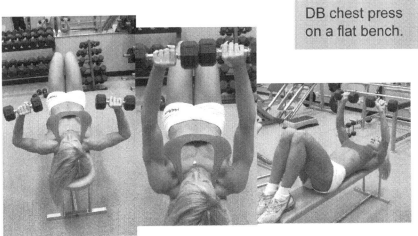

Training Program 2:
Resistance Training with Strength Bands:

30 minutes of resistance training. Work out two times per week. Perform 5 exercises that train the entire body. 1 to 3 sets of each exercise, 15 to 20 repetitions per set.

EXERCISE LIST:
Chest press or fly.
Standing rows.
Tricep extensions.
Squats. (either kind)
One arm chest crossover.

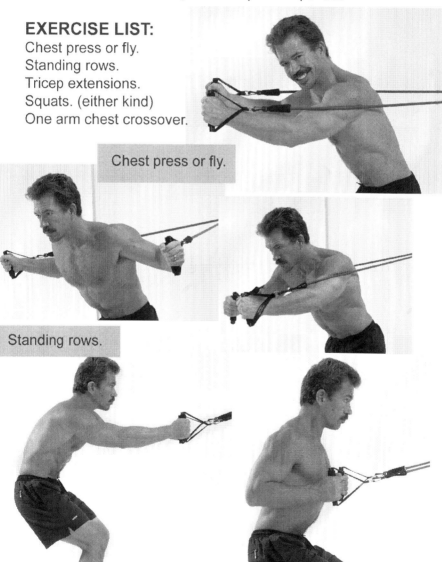

Chest press or fly.

Standing rows.

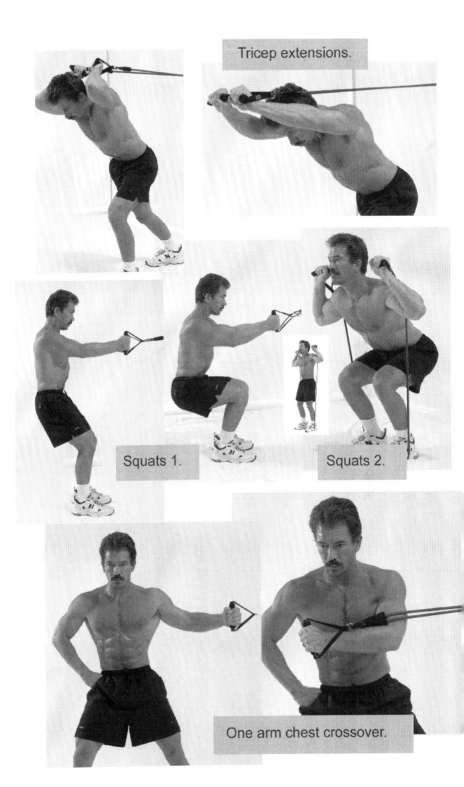

Tricep extensions.

Squats 1.

Squats 2.

One arm chest crossover.

Training Program 3:

Resistance Training with Weights:

30 minutes of resistance training. Work out two times per week. Perform 6 exercises that train the entire body. 1 to 3 sets of each exercise, 15 to 20 repetitions per set.

EXERCISE LIST:
Ab crunches.
On floor leg raises.
Single DB squats.
DB lunges on step bench.
DB chest fly.
DB shoulder press.

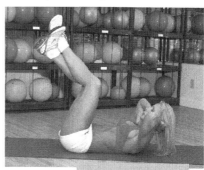

Ab crunches.

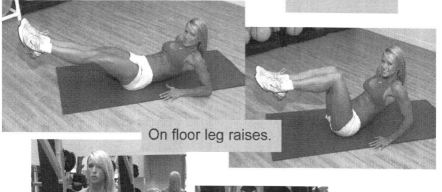

On floor leg raises.

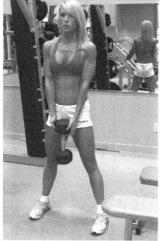

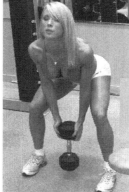

Single DB squats.

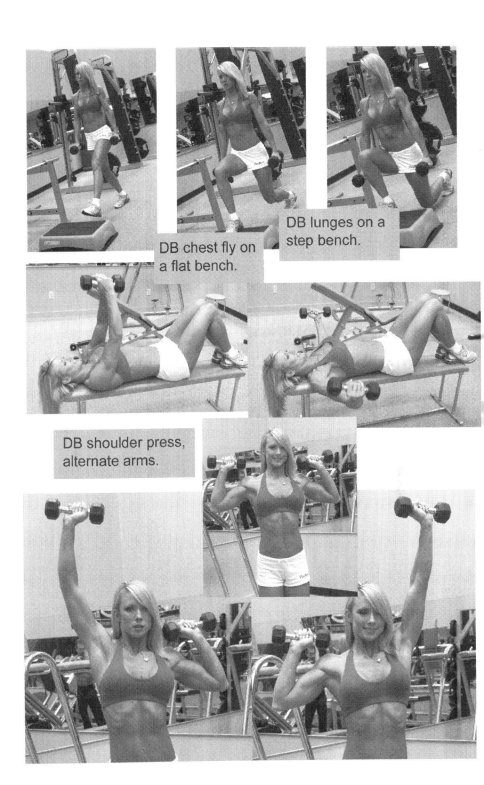

DB lunges on a step bench.

DB chest fly on a flat bench.

DB shoulder press, alternate arms.

Training Program 4:

30 minutes of resistance training. Work out two times per week. Perform 8 exercises that train the entire body. 1 to 3 sets of each exercise, 15 to 20 repetitions per set.

EXERCISE LIST:
Leg raises on leg raise station.
Sit ups.
Smith machine squats.
Leg extensions.
Leg curls.
Hammer row machine.
Hammer chest press.
DB bicep curls.

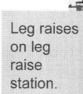

Leg raises on leg raise station.

Sit ups.

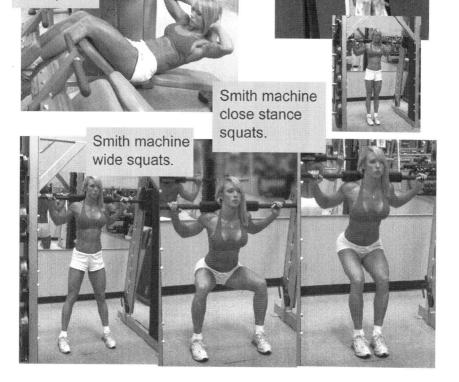

Smith machine close stance squats.

Smith machine wide squats.

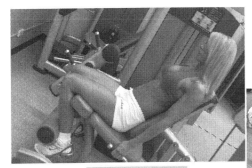

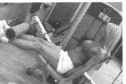

Leg extensions.

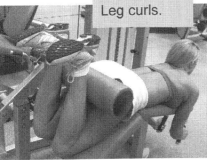

Leg curls.

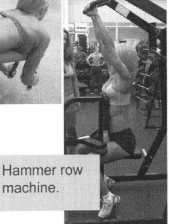

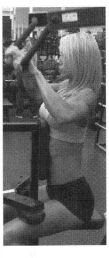

Hammer row machine.

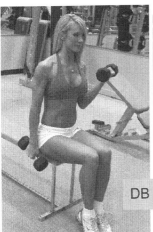

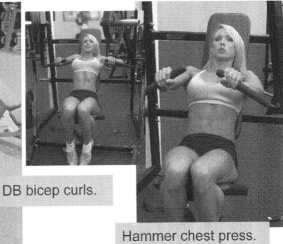

DB bicep curls.

Hammer chest press.

Training Program 5:

Resistance Training with Machines:

30 minutes of resistance training. Work out two times per week. Perform 7 exercises that train the entire body. 1 to 3 sets of each exercise, 15 to 20 repetitions per set.

EXERCISE LIST:
Slant board leg raises.
Leg press (close).
Leg press (wide).
One legged leg press.
Dip machine.
Lat pulldowns.
Seated pulley rows.
Bicep machine curls.
Tricep extensions.

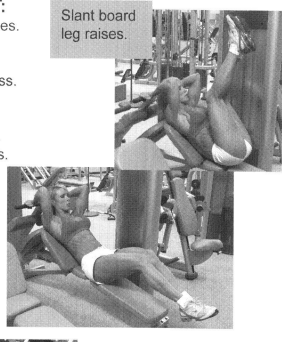

Slant board leg raises.

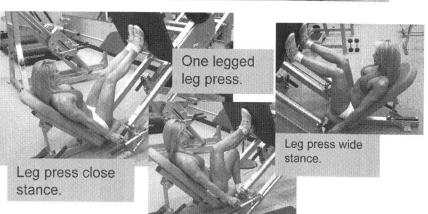

One legged leg press.

Leg press wide stance.

Leg press close stance.

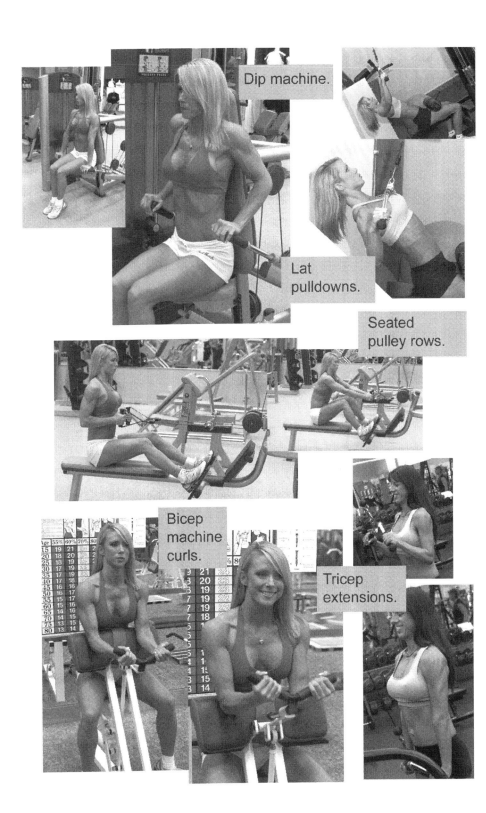

Dip machine.

Lat
pulldowns.

Seated
pulley rows.

Bicep
machine
curls.

Tricep
extensions.

Training Program 6:

Resistance Training with Machines:

30 minutes of resistance training. Work out two times per week. Perform 7 exercises that train the entire body. 1 to 3 sets of each exercise, 15 to 20 repetitions per set.

EXERCISE LIST:
Smith machine lunges.
Sit ups.
Slant board leg raises.
Hyper extensions.
Chest press machine.
Rowing machine.
Lower back machine.

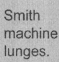
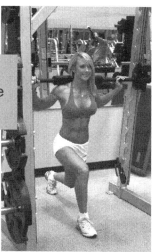

Smith machine lunges.

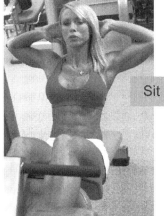
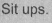

Sit ups.

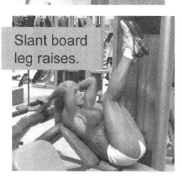

Slant board leg raises.

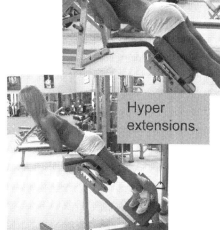

Hyper extensions.

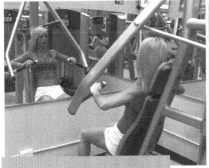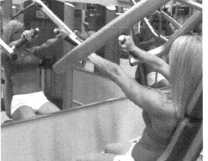

Chest press machine.

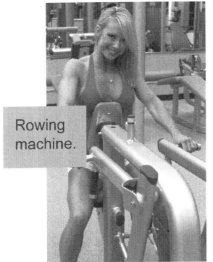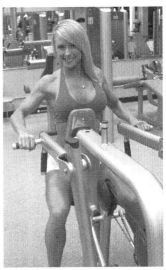

Rowing machine.

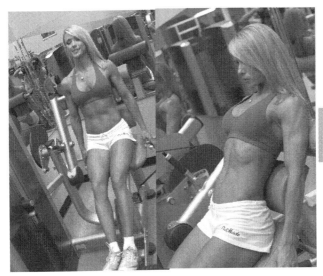

Lower back machine.

Training Program 7:

Ab Training Special:

30 minutes of resistance training. Work out two times per week. Perform 6 exercises that train the entire body. 1 to 3 sets of each exercise,15 to 20 repetitions per set.

EXERCISE LIST:
Ball ab sit ups.
Leg pullups on the floor.
Slant board leg raises.
Ball sit ups.
Torso twists.
Bench leg raises.
Ab bridge.
On floor leg raises.

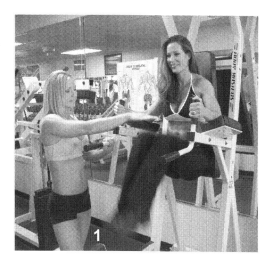

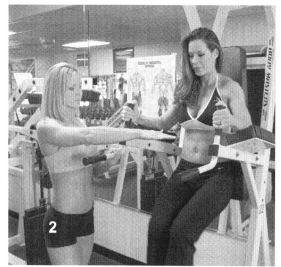

Ab station
leg raises.

exercise 1

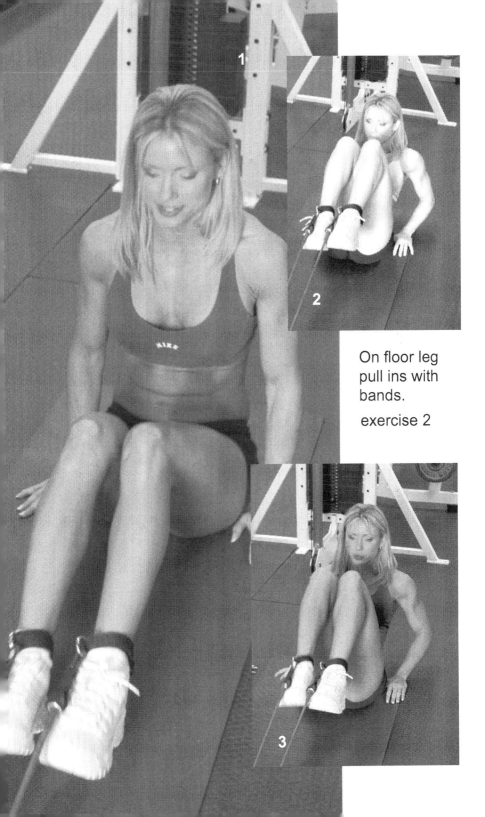

On floor leg pull ins with bands.

exercise 2

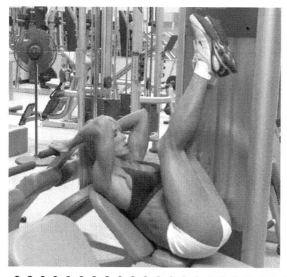

Slant board
leg raises.

exercise 3

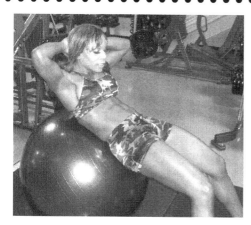

Ball sit ups.

exercise 4

Torso twist with
bands.

exercise 5

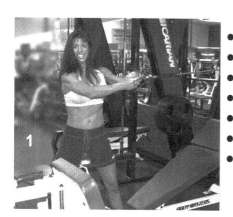

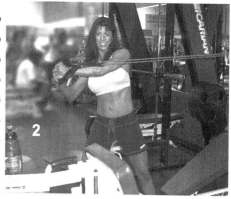

Bench leg raises.

exercise 6

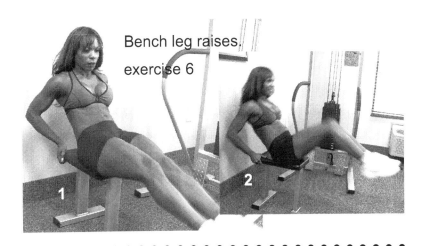

On floor ab bridge. Hold for 30 seconds.

exercise 7

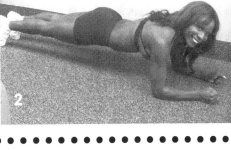

On floor leg raises.

exercise 8

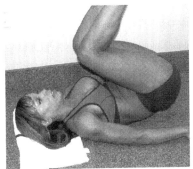

the
bi**k**ini
competition
training
guide

Training Program 8:

Butt Training Special:

3x a week

resistance training for the butt. Work up to 100 wide squats. Work up to 25 ball thrusts per leg, 2 sets.

EXERCISE LIST:

Super wide squats.
One legged
Ball butt thrusts
Lunges
Leg curls
Butt thrust machine.

One legged ball thrusts.

exercise 2

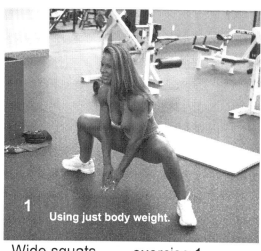

Wide squats. exercise 1

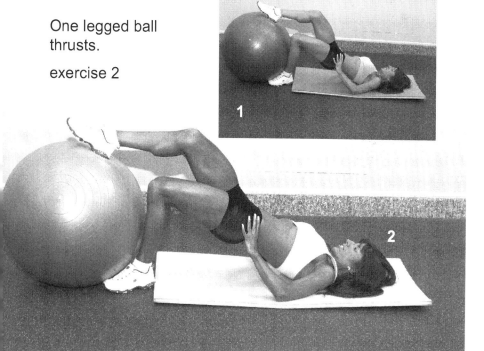

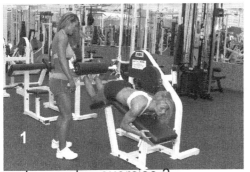

Leg curls. exercise 3

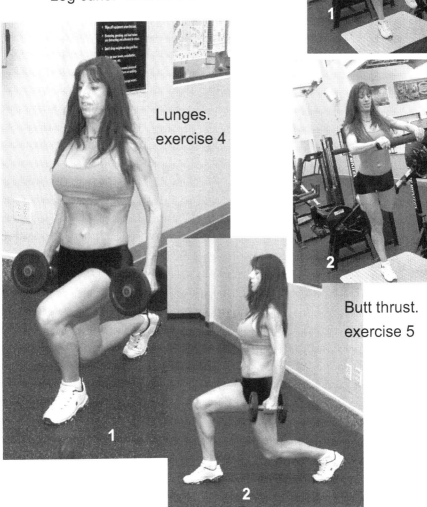

Lunges.
exercise 4

Butt thrust.
exercise 5

Split Workouts:
4 DAY SPLIT A

Monday	Day One
Tuesday	Day Two
Wednesday	Rest
Thursday	Day One
Friday	Day Two
Saturday	Rest
Monday	Rest

ABOVE: This is the most popular routine. You divide the body area in two, then train two days in a row followed by a day off. BELOW: Again, split the body in two areas but only train 3 days a weeks. This is a great split.

4 DAY SPLIT B

Monday	Day One
Tuesday	Rest
Wednesday	Day Two
Thursday	Rest
Friday	Day One
Saturday	Rest
Sunday	Rest
Monday	Day Two
Tuesday	Rest
Wednesday	Day One
Thursday	Rest
Friday	Day Two

DAY ONE

EXAMPLE ONE

DAY ONE	EXERCISES	REPS	REPS
Thighs	Squats.	3 to 10 sets.	12 to 20 reps.
	Lunges.	3 to 10 sets.	12 to 20 reps.
	Leg extensions.	3 to 10 sets.	12 to 20 reps.
Hamstrings	Leg curls.	3 to 10 sets.	12 to 20 reps.
	Stiff leg dead lifts.	3 to 10 sets.	12 to 20 reps.
	Ball butt lifts.	3 to 10 sets.	12 to 20 reps.
Calves	One leg calf raises.	3 to 10 sets.	15 to 30 reps.
	Two leg calf raises..	3 to 10 sets.	15 to 30 reps.
Biceps	Dumbbell curls.	3 to 10 sets.	8 to 15 reps.
	Biceps curls with exercise bands.	3 to 10 sets.	8 to 15 reps.
Triceps	Triceps extensions with bands.	3 to 10 sets.	8 to 15 reps.
	Dips on a machine.	3 to 10 sets.	8 to 15 reps.
Abdominals	Ball sit-ups.	1 to 2 sets.	50 to 100 reps.
	Leg raises on floor.	2 to 5 sets.	15 to 25 reps.

DAY TWO

DAY TWO	EXERCISES	REPS	REPS
Chest	Machine dips.	3 to 10 sets.	10 to 20 reps.
	Bench press.	3 to 10 sets.	10 to 15 reps.
	Chest flys with exercise bands.	3 to 10 sets.	10 to 20 reps.
Back	Front lat pull-down.	3 to 10 sets..	10 to 20 reps.
	One arm row with dumbbells.	3 to 10 sets.	10 to 20 reps.
	Seated rows with exercise bands.	3 to 10 sets.	10 to 20 reps.
Shoulders	Machine press.	3 to 10 sets.	10 to 15 reps.
	Lateral raise with exercise bands.	3 to 10 sets.	10 to 15 reps.
	Bent-over lateral raises with dumbbells.		

There are many ways to structure a split workout. Here is an example
of splitting your body into 2 parts.

DAY ONE   EXAMPLE TWO

DAY ONE	EXERCISES	SETS	REPS
Thighs	Smith machine squats.	3 to 10 sets.	12 to 20 reps.
	Front kick with exercise bands.	3 to 10 sets.	12 to 20 reps.
	Rear kicks with exercise bands.	3 to 10 sets.	12 to 20 reps.
Hamstrings	Leg curls.	3 to 10 sets..	12 to 20 reps.
	One leg band leg curls.	3 to 10 sets.	12 to 20 reps.
	Ball butt lifts.	3 to 10 sets.	12 to 20 reps.
Calves	Seated calf raises.	3 to 10 sets.	15 to 30 reps.
	Two leg calf raises.	3 to 10 sets.	15 to 30 reps.
Shoulders	Dumbbell press.	3 to 10 sets.	8 to 15 reps.
	Lateral raises.	3 to 10 sets.	8 to 15 reps.
Triceps	Dumbbell extension.	3 to 10 sets.	8 to 15 reps.
	Bench dip.	3 to 10 sets.	8 to 15 reps.
Abdominals	Crunches.	1 to 2 sets.	50 to 100 reps.
	Twists with exercises bands.	2 to 5 sets.	15 to 25 reps.

DAY TWO

DAY TWO	EXERCISES	SETS	REPS
Chest	Machine dips.	3 to 10 sets.	10 to 20 reps.
	Bench press.	3 to 10 sets.	10 to 15 reps.
	Chest flys with exercise bands.	3 to 10 sets.	10 to 20 reps.
Back	Front lat pull-down.	3 to 10 sets..	10 to 20 reps.
	One arm row with dumbbells.	3 to 10 sets.	10 to 20 reps.
	Seated rows with exercise bands.	3 to 10 sets.	10 to 20 reps.
Biceps	Machine Curls.	3 to 10 sets.	10 to 15 reps.
	Dumbbell curls.	3 to 10 sets.	10 to 15 reps.

There are many ways to structure a split workout. Here is an example
of splitting your body into 2 parts.

DAY ONE   EXAMPLE THREE

DAY ONE	EXERCISES	SETS	REPS
Thighs	Squats.	3 to 10 sets.	12 to 20 reps.
	Lunges.	3 to 10 sets.	12 to 20 reps.
	Leg extensions.	3 to 10 sets.	12 to 20 reps.
Hamstrings	Leg curls.	3 to 10 sets.	12 to 20 reps.
	Stiff leg dead lifts.	3 to 10 sets.	12 to 20 reps.
	Ball butt lifts.	3 to 10 sets.	12 to 20 reps.
Calves	One leg calf raises.	3 to 10 sets.	15 to 30 reps.
	Two leg calf raises.	3 to 10 sets.	15 to 30 reps.
Abdominals	Ball sit-ups.	1 to 2 sets.	50 to 100 reps.
	Leg raises on floor.	2 to 5 sets.	15 to 25 reps.

DAY TWO

DAY TWO	EXERCISES	SETS	REPS
Chest	Machine dips.	3 to 10 sets.	10 to 20 reps.
	Bench press.	3 to 10 sets.	10 to 15 reps.
	Chest flys with exercise bands.	3 to 10 sets.	10 to 20 reps.
Back	Front lat pull-down.	3 to 10 sets..	10 to 20 reps.
	One arm row with dumbbells.	3 to 10 sets.	10 to 20 reps.
	Seated rows with exercise bands	3 to 10 sets.	10 to 20 reps.
Shoulders	Machine press.	3 to 10 sets.	10 to 15 reps.
	Lateral raise with exercise bands.	3 to 10 sets.	10 to 15 reps.
	Bent-over lateral raises with dumbbells.		
Biceps	Dumbbell curls.	3 to 10 sets.	10 to 15 reps.
	Biceps curls with exercise bands.	3 to 10 sets.	10 to 15 reps.
Triceps	Triceps extensions with bands.	3 to 10 sets.	10 to 15 reps.
	Dips on a machine.	3 to 10 sets.	10 to 15 reps.
	Triceps extensions with rope.	3 to 10 sets.	10 to 15 reps.

There are many ways to structure a split workout. Here is an example
of a Bikini training body focused schedule.

DAY ONE   EXAMPLE FOUR

DAY ONE	EXERCISES	SETS	REPS
Thighs	Wide squats with light weights.	3 to 10 sets.	15 to 30 reps.
	Lunges.	3 to 10 sets.	12 to 20 reps.
	Step up on high bench.	3 to 10 sets.	12 to 20 reps.
Hamstrings	Leg curls.	3 to 10 sets..	12 to 20 reps.
	Kick backs with bands.	3 to 10 sets.	12 to 20 reps.
	Ball butt lifts.	3 to 10 sets.	12 to 20 reps.
Calves	One leg calf raises.	3 to 10 sets.	15 to 30 reps.
	Two leg calf raises.	3 to 10 sets.	15 to 30 reps.
Abdominals	Ball sit-ups.	1 to 2 sets.	50 to 100 reps.
	Leg raises on floor.	2 to 5 sets.	50 to 100 reps.

DAY TWO

DAY TWO	EXERCISES	SETS	REPS
Abdominals	Ball sit-ups.	1 to 3 sets.	50 to 100 reps.
	Leg raises on floor.	1 to 3 sets.	50 to 100 reps
	Hanging leg raises.	1 to 3 sets.	50 to 100 reps.
Back	Front lat pull-down.	1 to 2 sets..	10 to 20 reps.
	One arm row with dumbbells.	1 to 2 sets.	10 to 20 reps.
	Seated rows with exercise bands	1 to 2 sets.	10 to 20 reps.
Shoulders	Machine press.	1 to 2 sets..	10 to 15 reps.
	Lateral raise with exercise bands.	1 to 2 sets...	10 to 15 reps.
	Bent-over lateral raises with dumbbells.		
Biceps	Dumbbell curls.	1 to 2 sets..	10 to 15 reps.
	Biceps curls with exercise bands.	1 to 2 sets..	10 to 15 reps.
Triceps	Triceps extensions with bands.	1 to 2 sets...	10 to 15 reps.
	Triceps extensions with rope.	1 to 2 sets..	10 to 15 reps.

There are many ways to structure a split workout. Here is an example
of a Bikini training body focused schedule.

DAY ONE   EXAMPLE FIVE

DAY ONE	EXERCISES	SETS	REPS
Thighs	Wide squats with light weights.	3 to 10 sets.	15 to 30 reps.
	Lunges.	3 to 10 sets.	12 to 20 reps.
	Step up on high bench.	3 to 10 sets.	12 to 20 reps.
Hamstrings	Leg curls.	3 to 10 sets.	12 to 20 reps.
	Kick backs with bands.	3 to 10 sets.	12 to 20 reps.
	Ball butt lifts.	3 to 10 sets.	12 to 20 reps.
Calves	One leg calf raises.	3 to 10 sets.	15 to 30 reps.
	Two leg calf raises.	3 to 10 sets.	15 to 30 reps.
Abdominals	Ball sit-ups.	1 to 2 sets.	50 to 100 reps.
	Leg raises on floor.	2 to 5 sets.	50 to 100 reps.

DAY TWO

DAY TWO	EXERCISES	SETS	REPS
Thighs	Forward kicks with bands	3 to 10 sets.	15 to 30 reps.
	Reverse kicks with bands.	3 to 10 sets.	12 to 20 reps.
	Walking in heels.	10 minutes.	
Hamstrings	Leg curls with bands.	1 to 2 sets.	12 to 20 reps.
	Kick backs with bands.	1 to 2 sets.	12 to 20 reps.
	Ball butt lifts.	1 to 2 sets.	12 to 20 reps.
Calves	One leg calf raises.	3 to 10 sets.	15 to 30 reps.
	Two leg calf raises.	3 to 10 sets.	15 to 30 reps.
Abdominals	Twists with bands.	2 to 5 sets.	50 to 100 reps.
	Leg raises in ab station.	2 to 5 sets.	50 to 100 reps.

Aerobic (cardio) Training Schedules:

	MONDAY	TUESDAY	WEDNESDAY	THURSDAY	FRIDAY	SATURDAY	SUNDAY
BEGINNER	15 to 30 minutes aerobics	Rest.	15 to 30 minutes aerobics	Rest.	Rest.	15 to 30 minutes aerobics	15 to 30 minutes aerobics
INTERMEDIATE	30 minutes aerobics	Rest.	30 minutes aerobics	30 minutes aerobics	Rest.	30 minutes aerobics	30 minutes aerobics
ADVANCED ONE	30 to 40 minutes aerobics	30 to 40 minutes aerobics	30 to 40 minutes aerobics	30 to 40 minutes aerobics	30 to 40 minutes aerobics	30 to 40 minutes aerobics	30 to 40 minutes aerobics

ADVANCED TWO

AM

MONDAY	TUESDAY	WEDNESDAY	THURSDAY	FRIDAY	SATURDAY	SUNDAY
30 minutes aerobics	30 to 40 minutes aerobics	30 minutes aerobics	30 minutes aerobics	30 minutes aerobics	30 minutes aerobics	30 minutes aerobics

PM

MONDAY	TUESDAY	WEDNESDAY	THURSDAY	FRIDAY	SATURDAY	SUNDAY
30 minutes aerobics	30 to 40 minutes aerobics	30 minutes aerobics	30 minutes aerobics	30 minutes aerobics	30 minutes aerobics	30 minutes aerobics

37. No Workout Dairy:

We know why we keep a training journal; it allows us to keep accurate track of our training programs and food consumption. But, (drum roll) what if (like 90% of most people) you don't keep a diary, what then? Is all hope lost to be a champion? Of course not!

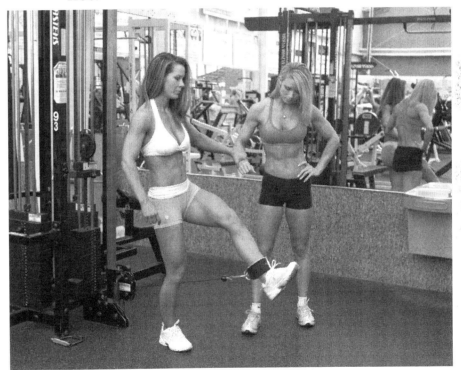

Can you make progress? Yes. As long as you gradually make your exercise routines harder, by slowly raising weights, increasing sets or reps, training longer. And eating a clean diet devoid of trash food that makes you fat. Follow the daily eating guides in this book and you will be eating clean.

Stick these basics and you will be a success in the your training and dieting.

Think of your training routine as a constantly evolving thing that is open to change at every workout. You must increase the intensity and duration of your workouts to make progress. Over time the central idea of training is to (slowly) increase the overall resistance, so that your body is forced to respond and become firmer, thinner, and stronger in response to the increased intensity.

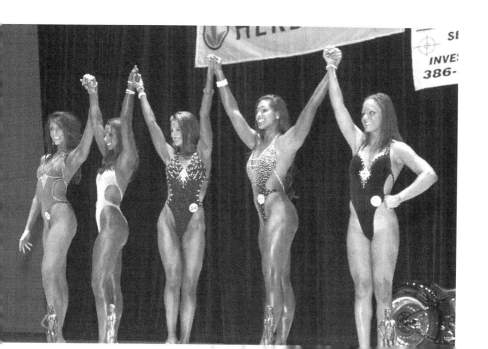

the
bikini
competition
training
guide

38. Sets and repetitions.

SETS AND REPS:

Warm up sets:

Each exercise will require some light warm-up sets to protect you from injury. Always warm up well on each exercise by doing several light sets.

Working sets:

Once you are warmed up, you can start adding weight to the sets, working up to your maximum workout resistance for that exercise. These are your "working sets".

Anywhere from 3 to 10 sets is good here. It all depends on how long it takes for you to tire out and how acclimated to training you have become.

BEGINNERS:

2 to 3 warm-up sets followed by, 2 to 3 working sets.

INTERMEDIATE:

3 to 4 warm-up sets followed by, 4 to 6 working sets.

ADVANCED:

3 to 4 warm-up sets followed by, 5 to 7 working sets.

BODY PARTS AND REPS:

Some body parts respond well to different repetition ranges and so on.

Ab training contains it's own special rules:

For pre-contest mode or if you in bad shape, abs can be trained daily for months. Abs can handle lots of repetitions. Ball sit ups working up to sets of 100 repetitions is a good goal for most beginners. High reps work well for abs. DO not train abs with weights. Some tension is good (like doing torso twists) but heavy sit-ups holding a weight disc are out.

Here are some rep ranges for the different body parts:

LEGS:

Legs respond well with both high reps and low reps.

The best is about 15 to 20 reps per set.

ARMS and CHEST and DELTOIDS:

The upper torso responds well from high reps and low reps.

The best is about 8 to 15 reps per set.

BACK:

Back responds best from low reps.

The best is about 6 to 12 reps per set.

CALFS:

Calfs respond best from high reps done slowly with lots of stretching and contracting during each rep.

The best is about 15 to 25 reps per set.

FOREARMS:

Forearms respond best from high reps.

The best is about 15 to 25 reps per set.

ABDOMINALS:

High reps with no weights.

The best is about 20 to 50 reps per set.

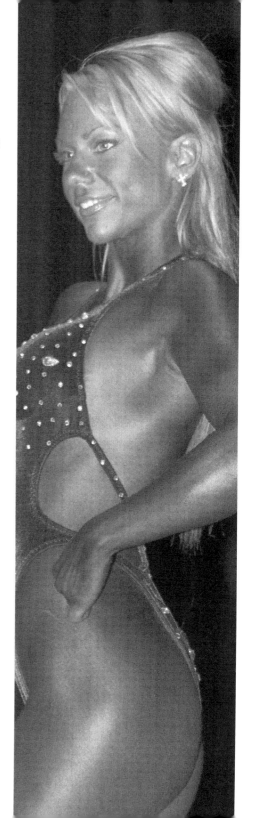

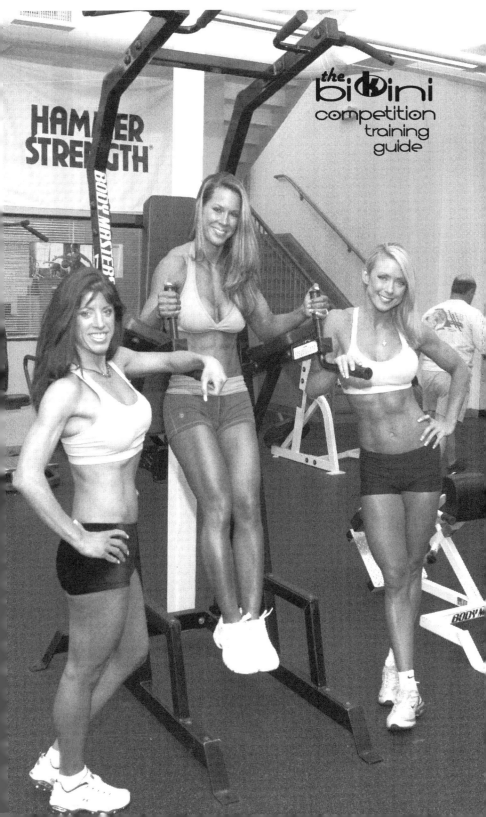

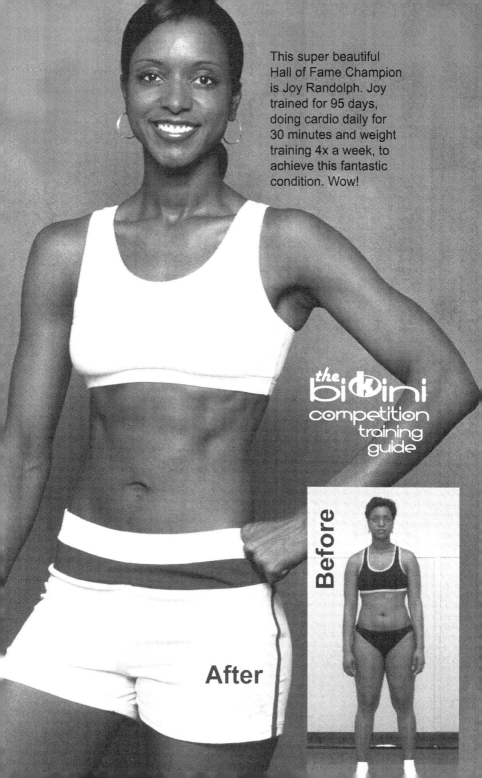

This super beautiful Hall of Fame Champion is Joy Randolph. Joy trained for 95 days, doing cardio daily for 30 minutes and weight training 4x a week, to achieve this fantastic condition. Wow!

the
bikini
competition
training
guide

Before

After

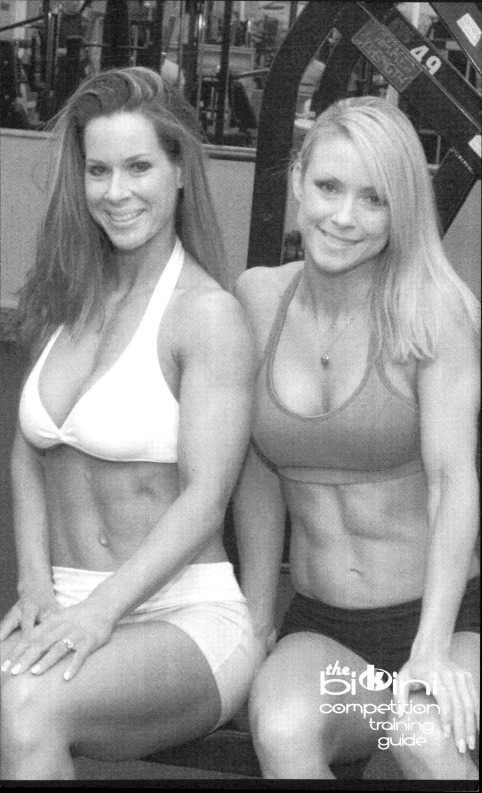

It Doesn't matter where you start!

Dan Burke in seminar.

It matters where you finish!

the bikini competition training guide

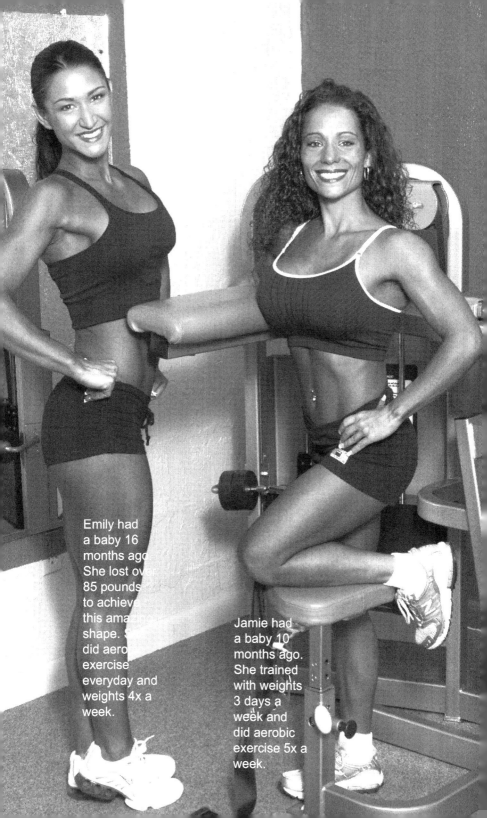

Emily had a baby 16 months ago. She lost over 85 pounds to achieve this amazing shape. She did aerobic exercise everyday and weights 4x a week.

Jamie had a baby 10 months ago. She trained with weights 3 days a week and did aerobic exercise 5x a week.

THE FIGURE COACH

Julie Green had
a baby 3 years
ago. Julie is
owner of one of
the world's fittest
bodies. She
trained 3x a week
with aerobics
and dieted for
over 6 months
to achieve
this fantastic
condition.

*F*inal Encouragement From Author, Dan Burke.

DON'T LOSE FAITH.

Expect to fail several times before you finally find the way to do almost anything valuable in this life. This includes riding the horse of fat loss. When you fall off, dust yourself off and get back on the horse. None of us are perfect. Seldom do we get it right the first time. My advice is, no matter what--don't give up on yourself. The real goal of being lean and healthy is so we can live a productive life and care for the people we love. Good luck.

Dan Burke

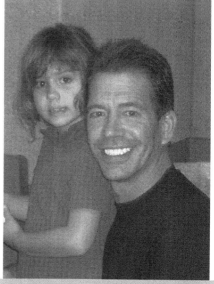

Dan Burke with daughter Lauren.

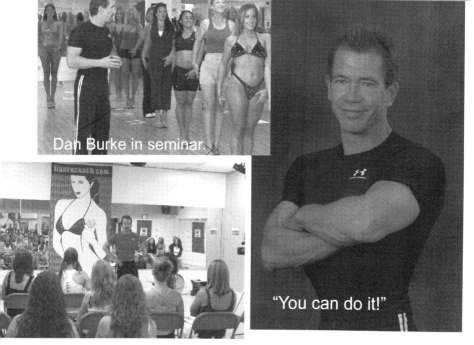

Dan Burke in seminar.

"You can do it!"

www.figurecoach.com

the bikini competition training guide

Amy trained 4x a week with aerobics and 4x a week with weights and dieted for over 6 months to achieve this fantastic condition.

Amy Bates

12118449R10113

Made in the USA
Lexington, KY
24 November 2011